Jessica Settergren
Foreword by Morgan Daimler

Defying Shadows

For Witches and Pagans Battling
Cancer and Chronic Illness

Chicago, Illinois

Defying Shadows: For Witches and Pagans Battling Cancer and Chronic Illness © 2025 by Jessica Settergren. All rights reserved. No part of this book may be reproduced in any manner whatsoever without written permission from Crossed Crow Books, except in the case of brief quotations embodied in critical articles and reviews.

Paperback ISBN: 978-1-959883-94-4
Library of Congress Control Number on file.

Disclaimer: Crossed Crow Books, LLC does not participate in, endorse, or have any authority or responsibility concerning private business transactions between our authors and the public. Any internet references contained in this work were found to be valid during the time of publication, however, the publisher cannot guarantee that a specific reference will continue to be maintained. This book's material is not intended to diagnose, treat, cure, or prevent any disease, disorder, ailment, or any physical or psychological condition. The author, publisher, and its associates shall not be held liable for the reader's choices when approaching this book's material. The views and opinions expressed within this book are those of the author alone and do not necessarily reflect the views and opinions of the publisher.

Published by:
Crossed Crow Books, LLC
6934 N Glenwood Ave, Suite C
Chicago, IL 60626
www.crossedcrowbooks.com

Printed in the United States of America.
IBI

Defying Shadows

For Witches and Pagans Battling
Cancer and Chronic Illness

About the Author

Jess Settergren was diagnosed with breast cancer in 2019 after a routine mammogram and spent the following year living through many of the worst experiences common to breast cancer survivors. She has been a practicing solitary Pagan since 1996, studying Wiccan, Norse, Greek, and Irish traditions for worship, philosophy, and craft. She has been dedicated to The Morrigan since 2012 and was ordained in 2020. Jess lives in the woods with her husband and a horde of kids, dogs, and a cat who rules them all.

To Mom:
In all the best ways,
I learned it by watching you.

ACKNOWLEDGEMENTS

Thank you to my parents for driving me to endless appointments, sitting with me during chemotherapy, making dinners, reminding me to rest, and all the ways you've supported me during, before, and after cancer. Thank you to my sisters, Kate and Nicole, for support and encouragement; Elyse, for cleaning my house while I couldn't get off the couch and making sure I ate during the worst of the Red Devil; the Ladies Aid and G.W., for hand-pats, "fuck cancer" talismans, care packages, dog sitting, fuzzy stick-on eyebrows, hugs, laughter and tears, and a freezer full of meals. Thank you, Ben and Sarah, who never doubted and held up hope for me when I was too tired to hold it myself. Thank you to my extended family, both blood and not, who cheered me on, cleared snow off my driveway, shared jokes and memes and Reiki gifts, fed me, and kept me going online and in person. This book wouldn't be here if you hadn't supported me through breast cancer, because I wouldn't have made it without you. I love you all.

To *The First Rule of Pagan Club*, for your knowledge and suggestions, especially with stones and chants: I'm grateful to know you. To Heather, Whitley, Shawn, and Katie for

Tuesday writing group: you've made me a better writer and you made this book better.

To everyone at Crossed Crow Books: thank you for your patience with this nervous new author's endless questions, and for believing in this book. To Lee and Kierstin: I owe you both a giant hug (I promise not to make it awkward) for everything you've done for *Defying Shadows*. I learned so much during this process, and this book wouldn't be what it is without your help. I'm so grateful!

To my beloveds, Jeff and the horde (Milo, Marilu, Zona, and Zeke): thank you for believing I could do it, and for enthusiastically accepting a weirdo witch for a wife and bonus mom.

CONTENTS

Foreword .... *xiii*
Introduction *1*

PART I
DIAGNOSIS

1. PANIC **9**
   Mindful Breathing 14
   Beginning Meditation 16

2. DEITY AND LETTING GO **19**
   Meditation to Find Deities................... 25
   Ritual for Letting Go of Control 31

3. DIGNITY IN MEDICINE **35**
   Self-Support Ritual with Aphrodite........... 38

4. THE MONEY **41**
   Charged Coins 43
   Abundance Altar Charm 44
   Money Charm 45
   Simple Candle Spell for Prosperity 47
   Simmer Pot for Abundance 48

PART II
TREATMENT

5. FACING THE LONG ROAD **53**
   Ritual Offering of Hair. 55
   Ritual to Quick-Access Your Courage 63

6. PHYSICAL PAIN AND TRAUMA **66**
   Pain Relieving Ritual Bath. 71
   Basic Instant Lotion for Radiation Burns. 77

**7. PSYCHOLOGICAL PAIN,
   TRAUMA, AND EXHAUSTION** **80**
   Light a Candle Every Day 84
   Make Green Tea or Lemon Tea with a
      Good Dollop of Honey 84
   Meditate on Ways to Redirect Your Anger. 85
   Spell for Staying Positive While Throwing Up . . 85
   Find and Embrace Humor Where You Can 85
   Cuddle 87
   Connect with Your Body 87

**8. INCENSE, OILS, AND SCENTS THAT
   WON'T MAKE YOU PUKE.** **89**
   Courage Oil Blend 93
   Oil to Combat Nausea 94
   Other Oil Combinations to Try 94
   Base Room Spray One 96
   Base Room Spray Two 97

9. MAGICAL EATING. **100**
   Allspice. 101   Apple 102
   Anise. 101   Banana 102

Barley 102	Lemon 111
Basil 103	Lemon Balm. 111
Bay Leaf. 103	Lime. 112
Blackberry. 103	Mesquite. 112
Blueberry 104	Mint 112
Caraway 104	Nettle 113
Cardamom 104	Nutmeg. 113
Chamomile. 105	Oats 113
Cherry 105	Olive. 113
Chili 105	Onion 114
Cinnamon. 106	Orange 114
Cloves. 106	Papaya. 114
Coriander 106	Parsley. 115
Cranberry 107	Pepper. 115
Cucumber. 107	Plantain 115
Cumin 107	Pomegranate. 115
Dill. 107	Potato 116
Elderberry. 108	Rosemary 116
Eucalyptus 108	Saffron 117
Fennel. 108	Sage 117
Flax. 108	Tea 118
Garlic 109	Thyme. 118
Ginger 109	Tomato 118
Grapeseed. 109	Turmeric. 119
Green Tea 110	Walnut 119
Honey. 110	Wintergreen 119
Hops. 110	Yew. 119
Legumes 111	

Foods Recommended by Oncology 120
Prosperity Pancakes 121
Fortifying Lentil Soup 123
Low-Energy Marinara 126

Herbed Bread 128
Instant Pot Mashed Potatoes 129
Tea Recipes. 130

10. CASTING A VIRTUAL CIRCLE: ENERGY RAISING WHEN YOU HAVE NONE 132
Circle Casting Shortcuts 134
Creating a Ritual Cord Anchor 136

11. TALISMANS AND STONES. 141
Spell Charm Bottle for Healing 143

12. ACCEPTING HELP 147
Create a "Yes" Talisman 152
Fire Ritual for Releasing Wrongs 159
Spell to Give Yourself Grace. 164

13. GRIEVING AND FACING DEATH 167
Simple Candle Magic Spell for Acceptance 173

PART III
SURVIVORSHIP AND REBIRTH

14. CELEBRATING. 179
Ritual of Gratitude 181

15. LIVING WITH FEAR. 184
Expanded Breath Work 187
Focus on Five Senses Exercise 189

16. ONGOING TREATMENTS 190
Daily Check-In Ritual 192

17. THE NEW NORMAL 194

APPENDIX: CELEBRATING THE WHEEL..........201
Samhain 201
Yule................................. 205
Imbolc 212
Ostara/Spring Equinox.................. 217
Beltane 222
Midsummer/Litha 227
Lughnasadh/Lammas.................... 229
Mabon 232

Bibliography and Resources *237*
Cancer Resources........................*239*
Index *240*

Foreword

If the world were a perfect place, then life would be easy and pleasant. We would enjoy every aspect of it, no one would get sick and no one would suffer. If witchcraft was a panacea that let us have absolute control over everything, then we would only have to chant a spell or burn a candle and all our problems would vanish. But the world isn't perfect, and witchcraft isn't an instant solution to every problem. Life is messy and painful, and witchcraft is a tool to address various situations, but it doesn't remove the mess or the pain. It does, however, give us a sense of control and allow us to help ourselves in deeper ways. That aspect is what this book is about: not the false hope of a "magic" cure, but the real hope that comes with a set of exercises, mediations, and magical options that can support you through a difficult time.

Whether or not we each like to admit it, life is a chancy, uncertain thing. None of us are guaranteed good health, an able body, or safety from injuries. Many of us are dealing with or have dealt with serious health issues and most of the rest of us will at some point in our lives. We will likely face this same gauntlet of diagnosis, treatment, and recovery, whether it is cancer or something else, and find, as Jessica Settergren did, that most of the faith-based books, groups, and therapists out there are not designed for Pagans or witches. They may even be antithetical to Pagan spirituality or witchcraft practices. This can add to the feelings of loneliness and alienation that a life-changing diagnosis brings and can make the struggle to work through things harder. When we are struggling, hurting, and afraid, sometimes what we need most is a community who understands what that feels like and who understands that instead of praying a rosary, we light a candle for healing. That community isn't always possible in person or online, but through the medium of text, this book offers that same sense of community, that understanding, that comfort. It reminds us that, however alone we might feel as witches handling a difficult diagnosis and fighting through a devastating illness, there are other people just like us out there who have done what we are doing, who know the power of a candle lit with intention or a stone carried for a purpose.

Part autobiography and part witchcraft guidebook, *Defying Shadows* speaks to people going through cancer treatment, but it also speaks to those dealing with other chronic health concerns. While the personal anecdotes are very specific to one diagnosis, the suggestions and advice is broadly useful; it certainly resonated with me as someone who has struggled since my teens with both debilitating hemiplegic migraines and PTSD. The stories shared about Jessica's feelings about facing the reality of death while struggling to live resonated with me as someone who once almost died from a medical complication and had nothing to get me through but prayer and witchcraft. This book is far more universal than it might appear and can be valuable far beyond its intended audience. It is layered with lessons on living, facing death, and enduring.

Being ill, chronically or acutely, can be and often is a life-changing experience. It shatters our understanding of both the world around us and ourselves, reshapes our community, and, for many people, breaks the basic trust we operate under: if we just do the right things, we can control our health and our bodies. Cancer is a great equalizer. It doesn't care about age or attitude and, in many cases, doesn't care about lifestyle choices; it is something that can happen to anyone. In the same way, many other types of illnesses and injuries tear down our sense of security and control to leave us floundering. This is where faith can come in, as with the rituals to deities like Aphrodite or the Morrigan you will find in this book, and, for a witch, where magic can come in—not always the big dramatic magic of the movies or popular TV shows, but the daily magic of meditations and small spells, and the vital magic that is self-care. It can be as subtle as whispered prayers during crisis periods or as elaborate as complex rituals, but it helps us find a sense of control amid the chaos and fuels a feeling of possibility even in dark times. Witchcraft, at its heart, is and always has been about empowering people who have no power in their daily lives, and it is perfectly applied to health struggles when we might feel especially powerless.

The magic of healing the mind and body is woven through this book, but the most valuable healing is less overt. It is that magic that offers help when we are feeling helpless: charms for money, charms for courage, charms to have compassion for ourselves. It is the magic of sharing and experiencing her journey with her, the lows and the lower lows as well as the triumphs. The anger, the betrayal, the grief. We empathize and feel as if we are being empathized with, a beautiful gift of connection during a time and health battle that is inherently disconnecting. This is a 200-page conversation whose ending feels like just another beginning.

Dealing with a massive health challenge will always be a personal thing—an isolating thing—because only we know what our body is actually going through from the inside, so it's essential to be reminded that we aren't as alone as we might feel. Other people do understand, and beyond that, our spirituality is there to support us.

Facing illness and the possibility of death is terrifying, but it's good to remember that even when we feel the most alone, we never really are. We are surrounded by spirits and deities who are with us even in our darkest times. We have our own power even when we feel the least powerful. No matter how isolated we might feel, there are other people fighting the same fight, experiencing the same struggles, the same pain. It is so easy to forget all of that, unless we are reminded. We are stronger than we think we are, and so is our magic, which can help us not only literally (for those who believe in it) but also mentally. It can offer us a whole new array of tools to deal with what we have to face, as well as options we may not have considered. The real brilliance of this book is the way it looks at cancer treatment without flinching and says, "here are some options, don't give up."

Ultimately, like Pandora's Box, all that might be left is hope—but hope can get us through, especially when combined with some magical focus. Believing that we can endure and overcome what we are facing and that we can do little things to help ourselves is vital. That belief, the essence of hope, is what you will find here in *Defying Shadows,* amidst some very candid discussion of how hard being this ill really is and how hard fighting to live really can be.

Morgan Daimler

Introduction

I'm writing this with numb fingertips and toes. One of the less offensively undignified side effects of my treatment cocktail, neuropathy took the longest to appear and will, apparently, take the longest to leave. It's the uninvited party guest at your house who tagged along with someone else and awkwardly lingers long after everyone left, still blithely telling stories that are supposed to be funny but are only weird and uncomfortable while you're unsubtly cleaning up and just want to go to bed. Well, that may be a uniquely Minnesota thing: we're notorious for not being mean enough to just kick someone out when they have overstayed their welcome. Fortunately, there is no social requirement to be "Minnesota nice" to cancer.

Unfortunately, breast cancer does whatever it damn pleases, and evicting it leaves marks both seen and unseen. Some scars are visible: biopsy pokes, lumpectomy or mastectomy surgery, port placement and removal, radiation burns. Those are easy: the pain doesn't last long, and the scars fade, at least a little, with time. The average person wouldn't even see the burn scars in my armpit, just a slight discoloration. But cancer is more pervasive and insidious in the mind than in the body, and while doctors prioritize healing the body during active treatment, healing the mind and spirit is essential for survival during and, if you're lucky enough to get there, after.

I can't speak for other medical systems, but in my hospital, breast cancer has a finely-honed machine of support that (in my experience) exemplifies what this country's medicine *could* be for everyone. I can only assume this is the result of decades of the Susan G. Komen Foundation's marketing campaigns and October's various "save the ta-tas" awareness fundraising. That's how I was diagnosed; I scheduled my mammogram because the October pink/boobs/cancer slogans reminded me I was overdue. The propaganda worked exactly as intended.

When I started looking through the support resources available, I was struck by the sheer number of books, support groups, websites, magazines, and blogs out there. Most of them were at least partially religious or spiritual. Unfortunately for me, none of those support groups or prayer circles were from a Pagan perspective. There were some non-denominational (which too often means Christian bones underneath the repackaged "support" skin), and there were a few with a Buddhist, Jewish, or Muslim approach, but none were any flavor of Pagan.

I looked for books, because admittedly I'm not great at receiving support face-to-face anyway, and I hoped for some tips and tricks to read during my three-hour chemo sessions. There are *so* many breast cancer books. Personal memoir-style books, journey diary prompt books, medical and science-based books, religious books, gratitude books, save-your-relationship-during-cancer books, coloring books, even cookbooks specifically for cancer patients: search for "cancer" on Amazon and thousands of titles come up, a healthy chunk of them specific to breast cancer.

I searched every resource available to me for books that approach dealing with cancer treatment or cancer survivorship from a Pagan point of view. Amazon, Barnes & Noble, general Google searches, University of Minnesota, and public library searches—none had anything for breast cancer, cancer in general, or even critical illness from a Pagan point of view. I was disappointed. I wrote *Defying Shadows* in the hope it may be useful for others who need a book to refer to during their own journey.

For purposes of this book, "Pagan" is an overarching umbrella term encompassing nature-based faiths from an Indo-European starting point. Wiccan groups and solitary practices fall under Pagan when I use the reference, as do Eclectic, Faery, Norse, Greek, Irish, and other European nature-based traditions. My ritual tends to be loosely Wiccan-based (elements, quarters, and so on), but as I am not a part of a specific tradition, my practice tends to be more generalized. This book is only my perspective from experience; since I have no experience or authority in other paths, I would not presume to advise that this is the only way. It absolutely is not, and I hope that you adjust anything you find useful here to your own spiritual needs and background.

My background with witchcraft and non-mainstream religious faith has been a long, solitary journey. I've been passionate about mythology since I was about seven years old, and when I say mythology, I mean all religious parables and stories. I started on Bible stories for children (i.e., sanitized of any sex or violence), and found Greek and Celtic mythology in elementary school. It's probably not great for an eight-year-old to read about Zeus's various affairs and assaults in detail, but there I was anyway.

In high school, I started reading the standard resources on Wicca (Cunningham, Starhawk, Adler, Ferrer, and so on) and many that were not standard. I don't, however, identify myself as actively Wiccan. I have not been formally initiated, nor have I been part of a formal coven.

I've been an active witch for as long as I can remember. I did spells from horseback without realizing it and found God in the woods long before I decided in 1996, after moving out of my parents' house, to label myself a witch. I didn't know until later that the concept of "being a witch" reflects who I am, not necessarily what I do. I got there eventually.

I've been dedicated to the Morrigan for twenty years. I have served Her as a solitary Priestess for over a decade and have acted loosely as a Priestess in various ways for my community for nearly as long. I have neither led nor participated in a formal coven, mostly because my circle tends to be too individualistic for that, and because, to date, I've not been called to do so. I tend to be more direct and individual in my interactions.

I have also worked with Persephone, Freyja, Aphrodite, Frigga, Brigid, and others over the course of my studies and practice, especially during cancer treatment. Connecting with the Goddess of Spring who is also the Goddess of the Underworld was particularly reassuring when facing the possibility of death. I gave many tears to Aphrodite during the worst days of chemo, when I looked terrifyingly sickened and bald and wondered if I'd ever be attractive or loveable in this body again. I spent many meditation sessions in Badb's sitting room, talking about what would happen if I had surgical or chemo complications and died. Cancer hits where it hurts, in every unconsidered dusty corner and unopened drawer of life.

I am an extremely practical witch. My approach for this book is to be as direct with Deity as possible, because I simply didn't have the physical or emotional wherewithal to do fancy formal rituals while I was in treatment. I got pretty good at casting a circle from my bed and doing without candles or incense when the smell made me sick. I discovered the power of screaming "fuck you" into the toilet and feeling Her supporting me when I was throwing up for the seventh time on a day when I wasn't even supposed to have chemo side effects. I have never been a witch concerned with the right tool, the right herbs, or the right words for my spells and ritual, and cancer distilled that even more. It's possible that attitude makes me less "real" for some folks, and I respect that view, but I am the witch I am, and you are welcome to make changes to the material in this book for your own comfort. Any ritual or meditation I include can be adjusted to whatever level of formality you prefer, and of course you can add, change, or remove things as you see fit. I will include what worked for me as a suggested starting point, but the goal is personal meaning and connection for yourself.

From a medical perspective, I found out I was diagnosed with invasive ductal carcinoma of the right breast on October 18, 2019, at 1:37 p.m. Central Standard Time. Over the course of the next year, I had two biopsies, four ultrasounds, one uncomfortable MRI (this is where the concept of dignity left my life for a year, a story I'll save for later in the detail it deserves), one radioactive tracker injected into my breast, a lumpectomy, five months of chemotherapy, one month of radiation, and I'll be on a preventative hormone blocking medication until it brings on early menopause.

I had family support, friends checking in constantly, meal trains, gift baskets, movie nights, and someone with me for treatments, but I also lived alone. So, while the support I did have was wonderful, it was not constant. Even my mother, a retired nurse who came to every appointment, surgery, and chemo session, couldn't stop COVID-19 from locking visitors out of the clinic in spring 2020.

As it turns out, even if you have someone at your beck and call during cancer treatment, you are still experiencing the worst of it alone. Hopelessness and despair creep into your room to steal sleep in the dark of 3 a.m., tears come unexpectedly in the shower when you wash your hair and clumps come out in your hand, and insidious shame slithers and whispers nasty barbs when you physically can't let the dog out and have to call for help. That is the place where I hope this book can be useful, because a Pagan does not have to be alone in breast cancer treatment, even when we are adept at finding our own way.

This is not a medical treatment book and in no way replaces or suggests any alternative to medical cancer treatment. I'm not telling you how to handle your own treatment options, because that's between you, your Deity, your family, and your medical team. My experience has led me to highly recommend current Western medical cancer treatments: decades of research have gone into them, and science backs up oncology's advice. This book, much like some of the peripheral assistance offered during chemo (aromatherapy, massage, dietician consults), is intended to complement your medical team's treatment plan, with stories and suggestions on how to cope.

On that note, if you've picked up this book, it's likely either you or someone you love is going through a miserable ordeal with breast cancer or some other critical illness. Regardless of prognosis, this journey leaves residual emotional and psychological effects. I am so sorry you are going through this. I know it's awful. I know it's terrifying. I hope this book helps you find some comfort and strength.

Blessed be,
Jessica

PART I
DIAGNOSIS

1

PANIC

If you've read Douglas Adams's *The Hitchhiker's Guide to the Galaxy*, you know the answer to life, the universe, and everything is forty-two. I turned forty-two two months, eight days, and approximately thirteen hours before Megan, the patient coordinator at Fairview Breast Center, called with my biopsy results. Since my birthday that summer, I'd been making smartass jokes that for the next year *I* was the answer to life, the universe, and everything. As it turns out, that was exactly true; cancer forces you to put yourself at the center of everything, whether you like it or not.

In its own way, the kindly voice saying, "I'm sorry, Jess. It's cancer" in a sympathetic but matter-of-fact tone sets off a deafening bomb. It was a normal Thursday afternoon, just before my weekly 2:00 p.m. data mapping call with business customers and IT. The buzzing in my ears that started at "cancer" drowned out whatever Megan said next. I suspect she was quiet for a minute or ten.

Last winter, I tried to learn to ice-skate. It didn't go well; I spent a lot more time bruising my butt than gliding with any grace. Once, as I tried to stand up after putting my skates on, my uncooperative feet flew forward while the rest of my body tipped back and I landed on the edge of the bench, on my left side, just under my rib cage. I rolled off and lay on the ground for an eternity of seconds, unable to even gasp. I looked like a fish flopping on the dock, mouth opening and closing trying to inhale. My lungs were closed for business. It felt the same when I heard "breast cancer." I couldn't breathe.

I'd gone in for the second mammogram in my life earlier that month not out of concern, but because the whole "Think Pink" breast cancer awareness campaign reminded me I hadn't had one since I'd turned forty. I admit the propaganda guilted me into going; it was yet another thing to check off an already full October to-do list, and I'd seriously considered postponing the appointment. I had no history of cancer in my immediate family, so I was young and low risk and, by all rights, could've put off screenings until I was closer to fifty.

I wonder what my prognosis would've been had I waited.

The first post-scan notification was standard form letter wording, paraphrased into, "hey, we saw something and would like to do an ultrasound just to double check." Many people get that letter after a mammogram and nothing comes of it, so I wasn't concerned. I went to the imaging clinic for the second time that month and waited in the silly pink half-gown for my tech to be ready. (I'm a tall woman…that thing is an embarrassingly short crop top on me.) After I was called into the private room and settled into the correct position (lying on my left side, twisted so my right side was diagonal in the opposite direction, right arm over my head, like an awkward yoga pose), we chatted about normal things while she put cold gel on my right breast and ran the ultrasound wand over it. We pointedly ignored my nudity and the weird position, discussing horses and men instead. She had a very good poker face.

The radiologist did not. He gently said he saw something on the film and would like me to get a biopsy. The words made it sound optional, but his face made it clear it wasn't.

My first biopsy was at Fairview Breast Center in Edina, Minnesota, a different branch of the hospital system where I'd had my initial tests. The same ultrasound tech was in the room. I didn't know another ultrasound was involved in a biopsy, but I was happy to see a familiar face.

The next two paragraphs include descriptions of needles. Feel free to skip them.

Have you ever gotten an ear pierced at one of those mall jewelry stores that arm teenage employees with a little pink piercing gun? They line up the "sharp" tip of the earring to a purple sharpie dot on your skin, and you hear the *snap* of the gun going off before you feel any pain. A breast biopsy gun is not unlike that setup, except it's not pink (thank Goddess, because by that time I was thoroughly sick of thinking pink), and instead of an earring, there's a hollow needle loaded like a spear and wielded by an actual doctor, not a sixteen-year-old. Presumably, since an ultrasound monitor is used to find the tumor, the placement of the sharpie dot was also more accurate.

So, once the path was identified on screen and the dot was on my skin, the doctor gave me a numbing shot. The lidocaine sting hurt more than the actual biopsy. There is a boatload of pain, discomfort, and indignity involved in breast cancer treatment, but while the body position and nudity are both uncomfortable and undignified, the biopsy itself truly wasn't painful. Once I was numb, I watched the ultrasound screen as the doc slid a guiding needle into my breast, using the ultrasound to make sure the end was at the biopsy site. Then I heard the *snap* of the needle gun and watched it dip in and out of the picture on the screen. I made the doctor and tech laugh when I said that looked exactly like the xenomorphs in the *Alien* movies, the ones with the second mouth that snaps out to bite someone. After the sample was bottled, labeled, and whisked away to a lab, they bandaged me up and sent me home to pretend I was living a totally normal life.

It took a week for the results to come back with Megan's call. I put my cell on speaker and set it on the desk before I dropped it. Megan's voice buzzed in and out between actual words and complete gibberish.

Invasive ductal carcinoma.

Murfmttsnt.

Surgical consult.

Laslkenaul.

"I'll call back with dates. Do you have questions?" I had none; I hadn't even heard most of what she'd said. My throat was too thick with tears to coherently answer. I looked down at the notebook on my desk: I'd taken more notes than I thought, including instructions to *not* (underlined three times, so she must have sounded adamant) look at everything available on the internet because a lot of it is garbage, but to stick to a few trustworthy sites. American Cancer Society and Susan G. Komen Foundation were the top recommendations for researching my diagnosis, which I'd apparently also captured when she'd rattled off all the statistics and details that I hadn't heard.

The call ended at 1:46 p.m.

I sat at my desk and let the tears come. My thoughts couldn't slow down, circling a central drain of despair. In that moment, I felt utterly alone and despondent.

I was going to die.

I hadn't done all the things I wanted to do in this lifetime yet.

And I couldn't do a fucking thing about it. I was so angry and terrified of what was to come, I just shut down in my home office.

Panic is a swirling maelstrom of emotional and mental wreckage that stops all thought. It can stop all action. While "fight or flight" is the commonly used phrase for how we respond to emergencies, "frozen in fear" is also a phrase for a reason. Sometimes, when your brain doesn't know what to do in a panic-inducing situation, it can default to freezing until the moment passes.

I participated in active shooter training once, led by my local Chief of Police. He told the group that the goal wasn't to stop us from being scared or to teach us combat, but to give us potential actions to take. Thinking through scenarios creates options for our brains, and once we've created a "road" in our minds, that path is available for our adrenaline-fueled fear-mode brains to travel.

When I heard the word "cancer" applied to me, there were no pre-considered paths available. I froze. The body's fight or flight response releases adrenaline in a flood, which causes the body to take shorter breaths and tense up. It becomes a spiral that escalates the extreme emotional state, and your mind can't stop coming up with all the ways in which a thing can go wrong. I don't know how long I sat at my desk, staring at my computer screen, sobbing. I know I missed that 2 p.m. meeting and all the follow up messages and phone calls from my team, until I could breathe and think again.

The most common tool to combat panic is to remember to breathe. Deep, slow breaths allow space between what your body is trying to get you to do (Run! Panic! Hide!) and what your mind needs to do to get you out of the situation (think, plan, and act). The following exercise was useful every time my body and lizard brain tried to get me to run away screaming or curl up and hide under a chair in the doctor's office. It can be done wherever you are and requires no special tools or energy expense. You'll notice throughout this book that many of my rituals and techniques are as low energy as possible, because a person in treatment for a critical illness is already using all their available energy.

MINDFUL BREATHING

Sit comfortably if you can. If you cannot sit or lie comfortably, unlock your knees, and roll your shoulders up, then back, then release the muscle tension so they relax and drop. Repeat the shoulder roll a few times, forward and backward, and concentrate only on letting the tight muscles relax. We all carry tension in our neck and shoulders, and fear is an instant muscle tenser.

1. Close your eyes if you are able and it is safe to do so.
2. Breathe in deeply to the count of five.
3. Hold your breath to the count of five.
4. Release your breath to the count of five and release any remaining tension in your shoulders and neck.
5. Repeat.

If you find five seconds is too long or too slow, try three. The key is to breathe in as deeply as you can: fill your lungs and let your belly muscles relax so your diaphragm can expand. Give your body all the extra oxygen it needs, and when you exhale, try to exhale fully until you have no breath left. If you can, pause for a moment before inhaling again.[1]

---

1 Important note: many who struggle with PTSD and anxiety can get into a loop of panic that feeds off focusing on breathwork, which results in exactly the opposite of this exercise's goal. If this is you, please know the breathwork described in any exercises in this book can be excluded. In the Survivorship section, I include panic attack exercises that have worked for folks in my community who can't abide breathwork.

If you can breathe deeply for a few minutes and release a little more tension with each released breath, your mind will clear enough that you can think again. Thinking leads to planning, planning leads to a clearer path forward, and a clear path forward shows you the next action to take.

From a spiritual perspective, I consider meditation a listening or receiving mode in contrast to prayer and ritual, which is an asking or offering mode. When actively listening, it's important to focus your attention on the other person, taking in what they're saying with their words, body language, tone, and gestures, instead of thinking about what you'll say next. In my experience, communicating with a deity is no different. I have spoken to deities in formal ritual through prayers of offering, gratitude, and request; letters written and burned; verbally as though they were standing in front of me; and even just as directed thoughts. Listening, though, is a different skill altogether. It is not just closing your mouth, but shutting down your need to respond, think and analyze, make mental grocery lists, or mentally replay a conversation you had earlier that day. Meditation helps build the skill of shutting off as much of the noise in your head as you can so you can hear, feel, and intuit the more subtle messages coming at you.

Commonly taught mediation practices including sitting up straight with good posture, feet on the floor, and shoulders back. One teacher advised me to think of a string that travels up from the bottom of your spine right up and out the top of your head and to sit straight and aligned like someone has pulled that string taut without leaning forward or back. This seated position provides excellent practice in aligning your body and allowing for deep breaths. It builds core strength and works well for visualization during grounding and centering exercises. If you choose this position, practice will make it more comfortable for longer periods of time. However, you are not required to sit in lotus pose on a pillow with perfect posture to meditate, and you aren't required to be still. I often meditate while walking through the woods, lying in bed, or brushing the dogs, because a little activity to keep my body busy helps my mind focus. Perhaps you knit or crochet, bake, paint, or lie in a hammock and listen to the wind in the trees for your best version of finding relaxed focus. I encourage you to do whatever version works best for you, because the key is to find what helps you focus on listening. I find the following steps helpful until you're used to the balance of supporting your spine without slouching while letting your muscles relax.

BEGINNING MEDITATION

Sit on a chair, couch, or the floor. Use a cushion (or don't) as you see fit. Cross your legs, as you are most comfortable and least likely to have your feet fall asleep. If you're on a chair, try to let your feet rest flat on the floor.

Support your back with a pillow, the wall, the headboard of your bed, the back of a chair, or whatever will help support your upright position.

Sit straight and close your eyes. Imagine a string that starts from your hips and pulls your spine straight, emerging from the top of your head. Look straight ahead so your head is set squarely on top of your neck, not tipped in any direction. The underside of your jaw/chin should be parallel to the floor.

Take a deep breath and pull your shoulders up toward your ears, then pull them back so your chest is straight across instead of curved in a slouch.

Release the breath and let your shoulders drop down, relaxed. They should be neutral now, not slouched.

Sit tall and straight, without specifically clenching your core/belly muscles. Sitting tall and straight will naturally engage those muscles for support.

Focus your attention on your breath without doing anything about it yet. If breathwork makes you anxious, focus on something else: the feel of the material under your hands, the sound of your heartbeat, the scent in the space you're in, or a particular painting or picture that speaks to you. The key is to find something you can use as a focal point and repeatedly bring your attention back to it.

Thoughts will pop in your head, and the more you practice, the weirder and more random they may be. Every time a thought pops in, let it go by turning your attention back to your preferred focal point.

When you feel ready, breathe in deeply and fully to a five count. Hold for a five count. Release for a five count, letting all the breath out of your lungs without changing your position. Again, if box breathing like this causes any additional panic, focus on something tangible using a different sense and just breathe normally until you can close your eyes. As you continue the deep breathing, pay attention to the darkness behind your closed eyes and listen.

From here, meditation takes different paths. Guided journeying begins here, as does inner shadow work that dredges up the icky things you've shoved down below your conscious mind and still must face at some point. But just floating in this safe, warm space within, without specific purpose, is where I listen best. Thoughts may intrude here and there: notice them and either wave them off into the darkness or let them float away on their own.

This space is where it's easier to hear if your Deity or guardians have messages for you. While it certainly is possible to hear an actual voice saying something to you, in my experience the messages come as a feeling, a sudden idea, or a flash of intuition. Sometimes there's nothing until I'm asleep later, and I'll have a vivid dream that sticks with me after I wake up. Sometimes there's nothing at all except the peaceful space I've created in the practice—after all, just because I'm listening doesn't mean any deity is required to respond.

I confess find sitting upright and meditating difficult, so I often do mine lying in bed. The trick to doing it there is not letting yourself fall asleep (although, if you can get to that liminal space between awake and asleep, messages come clearer and other skills like astral projection and lucid dreaming become easier).

Shutting off the noise in your head can be difficult, and it takes practice. Maybe you try to meditate for five minutes the first time and only have a moment or two of quiet space. Maybe you have none the first time. Practice expands that space, and so does trying different methods. If you're getting frustrated because seated or lying down meditation doesn't work, don't hang on to the frustration. It's counterproductive, and there are other options. Active journeying works better for some folks. For some, that sense of internal quiet is more accessible by silent prayer or vigil or focusing all your thoughts on the flame of a candle. Some find that mental quiet with long walks or hiking in nature, spending time in a sauna, or fire gazing. Find what works for you.

It doesn't matter how you get there. What matters is that you're finding a space to catch your breath and listen, because panic is a completely normal and completely useless response for breast cancer treatment. You'll need to be able to hear your options and make decisions, which means you'll need to be able to think, and no one can think while panic is in charge.

2

DEITY AND LETTING GO

It's worth noting that you are not obligated to apply religious ideas with witchcraft to your treatment. Witchcraft is not a religion, but it is part of many Pagan sects in some form or another. You do not have to worship a deity of any kind to do most of the rituals in this book; please remove or rewrite any part that doesn't fit your own practice.

Paganism in its various forms has exponentially risen in popularity in the United States since the 1980s, especially when the internet took off. I was a teenager in the late 80s and early 90s; the information on witchcraft and alternative spiritualities available for a country girl living twenty miles away from the library was pathetic. In my community, God was an entity found in the Lutheran church on Sundays. For clarity, I was not formally confirmed into any specific church or denomination. I was baptized Lutheran, but when I was about twelve, my parents decided Sunday would be a family day instead of a church day. I still went to church for the important extended family events, but I also learned that a person could find God without human-driven organization. That worked better for me than formal services because I was always more comfortable thinking of any deity existing in the land, stream, and animals surrounding me on our hobby farm. I filled my backpack with mythology, high fantasy, and whatever "New Age" books I could find in the high school and public libraries. By the time I was in college, I was sure I was Pagan.

I have loved watching acceptance for Paganism grow and thrive in the thirty-some years since those days, sending roots and shoots into almost every aspect of society from schools to politics to military to prisons. Calling someone a "witch" when I was in school was an insult, but now the witch aesthetic is popular enough to be mainstream. Becoming Pagan clergy can now be recognized not only by your own circle, but also by governments. Witches and Pagans are much more prevalent in American society (although overall still a minority), especially in my area.

Sadly, in my experience, that prevalence and support didn't extend to the Western medicine machine. To be completely fair, my first stop after diagnosis was a surgeon's office for treatment consultation. Surgeons, as a species of health care provider, have a reputation of thinking they're gods already (which may or may not be accurate), and they stick with the facts and science of excision (which I found to be completely accurate), which is a good thing.

My surgeon sat with me, my mother, and patient coordinator, Megan (yep, same Megan), in his exam room to review my options and his recommended course of treatment, answering every question we had. He was comforting and positive, and suggested this would all potentially be over in a few weeks after surgery and radiation, because at the time it didn't look like chemotherapy was necessary. As surgeons do, he stuck to the available facts and science of my disease, which is exactly what a patient needs from the person who is about to cut cancer out of you: surety, confidence, and a scientific approach.

I loved that my surgeon was certain, capable, and had no qualms about removing my tumor. I appreciated that he and the nursing staff were clear and honest about post-operative care challenges, and that surgery was only the first step in correcting the unwanted anomaly in my meat suit (my term, not theirs).

His philosophy worked for the surgical stage of my treatment plan, but both Megan and my mom said a good measure of surviving cancer treatment is "keeping a positive attitude." To me, that is a generic code for "having faith this will work out" and sidles right up to the general comfort of belief in a higher power running the show. Megan offered pamphlets and websites for support groups for cancer patients. Some were faith-based, some secular. The faith-based support was uniformly Christian. That's no surprise: statistically, the United States is still predominantly Christian.

When my journey moved from surgery to oncology, the treatment approach drastically changed from laser-focused on a single area to a holistic view of body, mind, and spirit. Standard chemotherapy plans emphatically include space for Deity in support. One of the patient intake questions at the clinic asked if I'm religious, because it turns out the long, terrifying slog of treatment that doesn't involve scalpels is so exhausting, awful, and disheartening that doctors encourage getting support from anywhere you can. The standard local support groups for women with breast cancer were again offered along with resources for counseling and the names of a few local churches.

As it turns out, a strong spirit is more necessary during chemotherapy and radiation than any physical support, because a patient who gives up is a patient who sabotages themselves in treatment. In the throes of chemo side effects, the desire to live and determination to keep going is the only part the patient can still control.

Please don't misunderstand my use of "control" here: everyone has the right to say how treatment progresses or whether it progresses at all. But once the plan is in place and you're committed to seeing it through, the "how, when, and where" of treatment is handled for you. It takes mental and spiritual fortitude to continue to show up. Keeping your spirit strong with the support of your chosen deity (or, in my case, deities) is essential.

There is no specific "anti-cancer" god, goddess, or other entity as far as I'm aware. There *are* deities who can be called upon to help you heal, according to their traditional descriptions. In the Greek pantheon, you could investigate Apollo, Panacea, Hermes, or Hekate. In Egyptian mythology, Isis is a good place to start. In Irish lore, Brigid is often associated with healing. Honestly, a list of gods and goddesses who could help during a health crisis, and the ways to connect with them, could be its own book. A Wikipedia search for "List of Health Deities" will give you an extensive list to begin if you're looking for a research project.

The thing is, asking for healing from a god or goddess with whom you haven't established any sort of relationship is less likely to be effective. Relationships—even with deities—are built over time. Are you more likely to help a person you don't know, or a person with whom you are at least casually acquainted? Any deity you already associate with would be the best place to start, but I strongly believe the universe is weird and unpredictable, sometimes to our benefit. If a deity you don't normally work with is calling to you, take the time to learn about them and listen. During cancer, all help offered to us is useful.

What does it look like when a god or goddess reaches out? Maybe in your research, their name repeatedly pops up until you notice it. Maybe you dream about them constantly, whether you can remember details or not. Maybe you just can't get thoughts of them out of your mind. Not all gods and goddesses are direct: some reach out with more subtlety, but if you have a sudden urge to investigate a new name, follow that instinct and check it out.

If you already have an association with a deity (or many), it's worth asking for help there first, even if they aren't known as healers. I started with the Morrigan not because She is a goddess of health or healing, but because I already had a longstanding relationship with Her. I've worked with Macha, Badb, and the Morrigan for over twenty years. But with some prompting and listening, I started working with Persephone and Aphrodite during chemotherapy, and I've continued with them in post-cancer survivorship.

There has been a lot of discussion in Pagan and witch communities about appropriation versus appreciation in the past twenty years, and it's worth addressing here. It's sometimes hard to know what the "right" path is to find and relate with a deity. In my experience, deities are not proprietary, so if you feel drawn to one, it's completely okay to follow that path and learn more about them. I do strongly recommend doing your homework, though: learn the lore, rituals, and particular preferences of your gods and goddesses out of respect for them and the cultures they come from, especially if that culture isn't your own.

Unverified personal gnosis, or UPG, can be powerful and useful in working with any god or goddess, and if you work something out privately with them that helps, that's wonderful. You may have better personal results with offerings, herbs, or rituals that aren't part of that deity's historically accepted mythos. That's between you and the deity in question, and is fine as long as you both agree on terms. However, UPG isn't the same as respecting the culture and lore of a deity and shouldn't be presented as "the way" for others. Appropriation comes in when you're claiming your way of worship is the right way, particularly if you aren't part of the culture the deity comes from, or if you're profiting somehow from the sale of something that isn't really yours to sell.

I am of primarily Scandinavian descent and live in the North Central United States. I have no authority to say my worship of the Morrigan is the right way. I don't have Irish heritage nor am I strictly an Irish Pagan, which is why this book isn't on Irish Paganism or specifically on worshipping the Morrigan. There are many resources and the excellent Irish Pagan School to refer to for that. What I do have is a responsibility to learn Her lore, customs, and rituals as best I can, which apply in my usual activities.

Since this book is specifically on what I did during cancer treatment, which deviates from my usual practices, I can only say that any prayers, messages, or rituals regarding the Morrigan, Aphrodite, Persephone, or any other deity during that time were my personal experiences. These are not "the way" to worship any deity I work with, only examples of ways I dealt with my illness with those who I felt could hear and help.

The Morrigan is typically neither soft nor fluffy: for me, serving Her includes a lot of difficult and harsh work. I needed to view this catastrophic change as a tempering of spirit, a trial by fire I needed to pass through to continue in Her service. Framing my next few months in such a way was a purely personal discussion between Her and I and should not be taken as anything other than personal gnosis. Her support would be invaluable as both a steadying force

I could lean against and the "get off your ass and get this done" pushing force I needed.

If you are spiritually minded, I recommend looking to your gods and goddesses first for assistance during this trial. Cancer is, in even its mildest form (Stage 0), a hostile invader that ruins life plans and terrifies a person down to the bones. Deity may not be omnipresent in American medicine, but there is plenty of space and need for the gods in cancer treatment.

MEDITATION TO FIND DEITIES

Materials:
- Candle(s): gold and silver to represent God and Goddess is preferable, but not required (a white or purple candle will also work)
- Matches or a lighter
- Incense burner (charcoal for loose incense or a cone)
- Mugwort (incense stick/cone or dried herb), for psychic/prophetic dreams
- Abramelin oil (alternative to mugwort)
- Journal/paper and writing utensil

There are so many ways a god or goddess can call a person that entire books have been written on the topic. For this exercise, I suggest reading up on some traditional deities in your heritage, or from a mythological cycle that catches your attention, to start. Even making time to research different pantheons on Wikipedia and make a note of those whose descriptions stand out to you would be enough to begin.

Once you have a short list of deities who sound interesting and you've read a bit about them, meditate on them to see who calls to you in the strongest way. Find a quiet place where you won't be disturbed. If you choose to cast a circle for this exercise, do so now. Light the incense and waft the smoke over your head: mugwort increases psychic reception. If you prefer not to use incense, you can use a drop of abramelin oil instead. No more than a drop (or just wetting a fingertip with the bottle) is needed: rub your hands together and pass your palms close to your face a few times, breathing in the scent.

Light the candle. Sit comfortably where you can see the flame and focus your attention on its light. Take a deep breath in through your nose, filling your diaphragm. Hold the breath for a moment before releasing it slowly, allowing your lungs to empty completely before you take a second breath. If your mind wanders and random thoughts pop into your brain, notice them and let them pass, returning your attention to the candle flame. Breathe deeply for three to nine cycles, releasing tension and settling into a quiet, receptive state of mind.

When you feel ready, look at any notes you've made of the attributes that spoke to you for a specific god or goddess. Are they associated with healing or medicine? Strength, like Thor? Death and rebirth, like Persephone? Are they in charge of war, or sorcery (or both, of course) like the Morrigan or Freya? What about that entity attracts you? Close your eyes and ask the god or goddess if they are calling you. You may ask out loud or in your mind, but the question is the same.

> *"(Deity Name), I feel your interest.*
> *Are you calling to me? I am listening."*

Then, let your mind relax and pay attention to any different or new feelings that arise. Note down anything that stands out to you during this listening time. Messages may be changes in feelings, sudden thoughts, or faint echoes of emotions. If they aren't for you, you may receive absolutely nothing at all.

Repeat this exercise with all the deities on your list. When you're finished for the time being, thank those who communicated with you, snuff the candle, and open the circle.

This meditation may take additional time or repeated sessions to discover those entities you may want to work with. Once you have names narrowed down, or someone has made themselves stand out in a way unable to ignore like repeated dreams, it's time to do your part of the work. Research that deity, discovering how they prefer to communicate in and out of ritual. Read their lore and identify whether they have important dates, herbs, animals, or astrological events associated with them. Spend time getting to know what you can about them, but also take time to ask them directly about what they're like. Consider some basic "getting to know you" questions that will help you connect with them.

- Do they prefer formal rituals, meditation, dreams, or another way to connect with you?
- What offerings do they like, and how often?
- What incense/candles/oil scents are associated with them?
- Is there a piece of jewelry you feel you should wear when you speak with them? If so, a ritual to ask them to bless that piece with their protection and guidance may be appropriate.

At its core, building a relationship with a deity isn't terribly different from building a relationship with a new friend: it takes interest, intention, and consistent follow-through.

Remember that just because a deity is calling does not mean you are obligated to accept the call and build a relationship. If something doesn't feel right to you, it's okay to respectfully end the association. Agency, boundaries, and willing association are essential to any healthy relationship, even those with a god or goddess.

It's worth reiterating that witchcraft doesn't require god or goddess worship, and it's fine to eschew the devotional aspects of this book if that's not your jam. Working with your own will and the universe's energies is just as effective, and there's no reason any of the exercises (except maybe the one specifically to find out which gods/goddesses are paying attention to you) can't be modified to remove the deity aspects of the working. Self-reliance can also be a powerful source of spiritual resilience.

I'm a stubborn person, but I come by it honestly. At one point Mom commented, frustrated, that I don't need to be "so damn stoic all the time," which is silly since I came by my attitude legitimately from both parents. She's used a cane for the past few years, but she does not need help, *thankyouverymuch*. Dad slipped on the stairs and broke his ankle a few years ago and tried to insist he didn't need an ambulance (an ambulance was both needed and called). Stubbornness and self-sufficiency are in my blood.

Since I was in college, I have found pride in depending on no one for anything, from money to security to safety. Losing control over what was happening to me while this invisible interloper turned my existence upside down was hell. I'd like to be a smartass here and say something pithy about it being…difficult, with all the weight of sarcasm attached to the word, but honestly it was pure hell.

The man I was seeing when I was diagnosed reminded me that treatment was an exercise in letting go. He wrote me a whole series of messages one night, in the darkness of 1 a.m. when terror overwhelmed me as I lay in bed. fAngus (my occasionally homicidal cat) lay on my chest, purring and kneading the same side my tumors had been on before surgery. Ragnar, my young German Shepherd who sadly was not walked nearly enough during treatment, lay next to me with his back against my leg, snoring his bear-dog snore. It was the night before my first chemo infusion. I'd already cut my hair off, I'd done surgery, I'd told people at work and everyone at home, and I'd started my medical directive papers in case something went wrong because the clinic wants to know if you have a do-not-resuscitate order on file well before you end up in the emergency room. I couldn't do anything else. While the darkness pressed in around me and I felt most alone, he sent me a series of texts that helped with the fear of not running my own life.

I saved them, despite no longer being with him, because they helped me sleep that night before I walked into the worst trial of my life. I was so unbelievably angry that I couldn't even rule over my own body's bullshit, and I said so over text. I didn't expect him to see it until morning, but it made me feel better in that moment.

"You went to the doctor. You didn't wait, you didn't hesitate, you were properly ruthless on your own behalf, stuffing your fears and going 137% full tilt at this," he immediately responded, which filled my dark bedroom with the specific blue light of an iPhone's text notification. Never have I been so grateful for that intrusive light. "What else is there to do?"

"Jumping out of an airplane is hard. Falling and being afraid in the air is easy," he said. We'd had multiple conversations about how (supposedly) fun skydiving is and how vehemently I refuse to jump out of a perfectly good plane. "You don't even realize that you already did all the 'stand up/hook up/shuffle to the door' part of this, and from here everything is literally downhill. You're in freefall and now *is* the time to be afraid, because at this point your medical team and technology are responsible for treatment, not you. But you got your own ass to this point. And after all of this is done, and you are done with all this bullshit, maybe you will do some skydiving after all. Because, hell, how could you be afraid of anything else, ever?"

For the record, I am now through chemotherapy and radiation and surgery and no, I still have no interest in skydiving. However, he did have an excellent point about fear that I now regularly remind myself of when I am taking on a new challenge. It doesn't always stop the fear, but it does help me get to the other side and act.

"The doctors and the nurses and the chemo and the family and your support group and me…now it's on *us*. You need to remember that, just like falling out of the plane, everything that happens afterwards is inevitable. It's up to you to do the next right thing, get to the next vitamin, the next appointment, the next round, the next toilet, the next crying and screaming jag, the next argument with the Goddess. Because it's like falling from the plane: you already jumped. The rest is just falling and floating to the next step until you land."

I carried that image with me for the next six months as I went through chemotherapy and radiation. Despite growing up in a nurse's household, I wasn't always great at following the rules of being sick. There came a point where I could no longer control the outcome: chemo and radiation were going to do whatever they wanted to my body. I had to let go and be patient with being the patient.

Cancer taught me how to let go of the illusion of control I held regarding my health, my body, and my life. The next nine months were about tactical (immediate) cancer battles, and any other plans I had in mind would have to be set aside until I had the energy and wherewithal to take them up again. Give yourself time and grace to settle into the new normal with cancer, because, until you're in treatment, you can't possibly know how you will respond to the cycles of drugs and infusions, and it's okay to let things go in the meantime and focus on this journey as much as you can.

RITUAL FOR LETTING GO OF CONTROL

Materials:
- Small cauldron or firesafe bowl
- A pinch of spearmint or savory, for mental fortitude
- Matches or a lighter
- Paper strips or bay leaves
- Pen or marker
- Water, preferably filtered
- Plant pot
- Potting soil
- Seed, seedling, or a small plant of your choice. This works just as well if you buy the plant and re-pot it at home if you don't want to start from a seed. A snake plant for tranquility, positivity, and good luck, or pothos (Devil's Ivy) for protection, resilience, and forgiveness, would be lovely choices and both thrive indoors.

Variation: You could also use your favorite herb, or, if it's the right time of year to plant outside, you could do this ritual while planting in your own garden. In that case, I'd choose a morning glory or pansy to plant, because they're both so wonderfully explosive and prolific in their growth over the season.

This can be done as part of a larger ritual or as a standalone exercise. In either case, set up your materials in a space where you can work comfortably. Close your eyes and take three deep breaths, relaxing your belly so your diaphragm expands with each breath. When you exhale, allow tension to flow from your body. Pull your shoulders up toward your ears, then contract your upper back muscles to increase tension and pull the shoulders back. Then, during the exhale of a deep breath release the shoulders down and let those muscles relax.

With your eyes still closed, let the worries about your diagnosis and treatment plan come to the forefront of your mind. Perhaps you're afraid of surgery, chemotherapy, radiation, balancing caring for your family while you're in treatment, or your job's response to your medical situation. Perhaps you're afraid of how your children will react to the news and to seeing their parent weak and needing help. Maybe you're afraid of long-term side effects, or that your body won't be able to tolerate what's coming with treatment. Maybe you're just flat-out terrified of death. The worries you carry are both unique to your life situation and universal to cancer patients, and the loss of control is especially scary. When you're ready, open your eyes.

On strips of clean paper or large bay leaves, write out as many of those fears as you can. As you write each one, say:

"I will do what I can, and let the rest unfold as it will."

Take all the time you need for this part of the ritual, and don't be afraid to cry or rage if needed.

Light the papers in your cauldron or fireproof bowl. Allow each one to burn to ash. If you are unable to burn them, you can also soak them in water. While the papers burn or soak, prepare your new flowerpot. Make sure there's a drain hole in the bottom. Fill the pot to about ¾ full if you're transplanting a houseplant. Add the spearmint or savory to the potting mix. Using your fingers, gently dig the transplant hole deep enough for the plant's root ball. Place the ashes in the bottom of the hole, then place the plant's roots on top of the ashes and fill the hole with dirt (add more on top as needed). The soil should cover the roots of the plant.

If you're planting a new seed or seedling, bury the ashes or wet paper about two inches into the soil. Use your index finger to poke a hole in the center of the dirt about one inch deep and drop in the seed(s). Cover gently with soil.

Water the plant thoroughly, or if you've chosen to use seeds, water gently (you don't want to wash them out of their new home). Set in a well-lit area in your house. A pothos plant or snake plant does not need direct sunlight, but a pot with seeds would like some more sun. At this point, you may close your ritual and, if you've opened one, close your circle. Be sure to eat something to reground yourself.

Letting go of the outcome isn't something we can do once and be finished: this is a process that will need to be revisited regularly throughout treatment.

Every time you attend to the seed/seedling, be mindful of how everything blooms and grows on its own schedule. Every growing and dying cycle is unique, and no one knows what theirs will be. Some of this journey just isn't up to you. Sometimes, growth comes during the times we leave things alone and stop trying to meddle. Overwatering a fragile seed will drown it, and you'll never see the glorious plant it's meant to become. By allowing your fears and worries to compost and feed new growth, you relinquish the need for illusion of control and allow reality to develop as it's meant to be. All you can do is nurture yourself, take care of what you can reasonably manage, and let the rest happen as it will.

Of course, there are responsibilities you can't just drop. Parenting, work, caring for your own parents and pets—they all still need your attention and energy, and it's awful to feel like you're failing when you can't do everything or be everywhere for your people. This is also where letting go and allowing your loved ones to help you as much as you can comes in. If people offer to clean, cook, handle kid pickup or drop-off, grocery shop, walk the dog, do the laundry: start practicing "yes, thank you," because it will be important as treatment goes on for you to have tasks taken off your plate. It will feel uncomfortable at first, and you'll be tempted to just do whatever chore yourself out of habit, pride, or expediency. Letting go means letting yourself be helped by your medical team, family, friends, and, if you lean toward the spiritual, your Deity.

3

Dignity in Medicine

In addition to your sense of control, cancer brutally strips away your sense of dignity. After my biopsy and diagnosis, I had to have an MRI scan (magnetic resonance imaging) of my upper body before my surgical consult. By that time, I'd been half naked with some nurse's chilly hands moving my boobs around for mammograms. I'd been squished in the machine, exposed to the ultrasound tech (multiple times), imaged, needled, and shot with a biopsy alien-mouth gun. I figured an MRI wouldn't be too scary, since I'm not terribly claustrophobic, but it turned out to be a whole new level of awful.

Let's start with the (always too-short) hospital gown opening to the front, an unpleasantness I was barely beginning to get used to, followed by walking down the freezing hospital hall from the dressing room to the MRI room in nothing but purple non-slip hospital socks, panties, and that thin fabric that does nothing to keep you warm in the icy temperature health care facilities prefer. I should say that I am generally far from prude: I spent twenty years changing into and out of costume in a Renaissance Festival parking lot every autumn. I discovered that even I have *some* limits when it comes to exposing myself to strangers. The MRI process was less than pleasant for my comfort level of bodily exposure.

The nurses went over the whole procedure with me in advance, I assume because a lot of people freak out about being in that noisy little tube. I'm six feet tall and stocky. The MRI tube is *much* smaller in diameter than I'd been led to believe from shows like *Grey's Anatomy* and *ER*. I was told I had to lie face-down, which I thought was great because I could just pretend that I'm taking a nap, until I saw the contraption I had to lie over.

A breast MRI is face down, but you don't get to lie comfortably in any natural position. The nurses have you kneel on the MRI bed on all fours over a frame that has two side-by-side open boxes with a two-inch-wide metal brace between. Your gown is open. Your breasts hang into the boxes, and that brace is where *all* your upper body weight lands, concentrated along your sternum. My upper body weight is significant; it is not a comfortable position.

Once your udders hang in the boxes (nothing is pretty or perky in the MRI room) and the center brace is digging into your breastbone, the nurses kindly cover you with a couple of heated blankets, put noise cancelling headphones over your ears, and insert you headfirst into the tiny tube. Since you're raised halfway up your knees, the top of the tube is only a couple inches away from your back, and you can *feel* that the top is too close. I kept my eyes closed to try to mitigate anxiety, but it rose as the process went on. If you're allowed to take Valium or something to keep you calm during an MRI in your treatment plan and you have even a smidge of claustrophobia, it's worth consideration.

The technician could talk to me through the headphones, and they asked what I'd like for music. I chose spa themes because my intent was to meditate. I should've chosen heavy metal: noise cancelling headphones don't cancel the MRI buzz.

The voice in my headphones popped in and out of the buzzing and music to keep me in the loop. They told me how long each imaging session will be before they started, and they checked on my freak-out-factor before and after each one. I had six sessions in that hellish position, ranging from thirty seconds to twenty minutes long. If I moved during a session, we had to start over. I closed my eyes and breathed as deeply as I could with all my torso's weight on that stupid box frame and tried to mentally go away.

Did you know magnetic resonance imaging has a physically tangible effect? Maybe it was my position because my back was so close to the top of the tube, but every time we started a session, it felt like ten thousand fairies marching up and down my back, tickling and dancing and wiggling the blanket. The box's brace against my torso felt like it was bruising my bones because I couldn't shift my weight. All of this was happening while my boobs hung in a box so the hospital could take pictures of them in the most unflattering way.

My MRI showed an additional smaller tumor, which meant another round of biopsy-wait-results time. Ultimately, I decided to get a lumpectomy, not a full mastectomy. My surgeon was confident he could get both tumors out and a lymph node from my armpit (to verify if the cancer has spread beyond the breast tissue), and I believed him.

Surgery involved another stupid gown that opens to the front, a nurse coloring on my breast with purple permanent marker, an IV given by someone who doesn't do phlebotomy enough to get it in on the first try, and a radioactive tracker.

Surgery also required a pregnancy test I didn't consent to. If you are a person physically capable of bearing children, it does not matter what you say: surgeons will not work on you without a pregnancy test. Never mind your partner is fixed, never mind you haven't had sex for a year: if you are still having a period more often than once a year, they force you to pee in a cup. It's just another way to cover their own liability and ignore your word. Honestly, it was a small question that brought out a whole slew of anger at the hospital and nurses: to this day, I am salty about it and would like to give the whole medical system in the United States the finger for removing a woman's agency.

At some point during all the awful medical procedures that treat your body like a separate entity, your dignity just gets left in the bin with the used front-open hospital gowns. When my two-week recovery check-up happened in a conference room at the clinic instead of an actual exam room, it barely occurred to me to close the window shades before pulling my tank top down so my surgeon could check the two incisions on my areola and one along the edge of my armpit.

In those first days after the flurry of tests, strangers poking and prodding me, surgery, and recovery, I found some solace having conversations with Aphrodite. I have a statue of Her in my bathroom, the most intimate room in the house where baths/showers are performed, where hair is brushed and makeup is put on and removed. She is the Goddess of Love I connect with the best, and who better to help me adjust how I think of myself so I am more grounded in my skin, even when faced with indignities from which I'd rather escape?

SELF-SUPPORT RITUAL WITH APHRODITE

Materials:
- Mirror, above a sink or in a bathroom with a tub/shower

Helpful additions (any of these would do):
- Statue of Aphrodite
- Half of a scallop shell
- A rose, for love (in this case self-love) and as offering to Aphrodite
- Floral bath oil/perfume, in any scent that makes you feel good/positive/happy

Note: If you have the energy and desire to do so, feel free to call the quarters and make this a more formal ritual. The general concept of this book is to offer rituals that you can do when you're not feeling up to anything, so please know you can add whatever formality you need as you like.

If you are allowed to do so, take a ritual bath or shower. You can add some scented oil you like to the tub or shower if you like. Take a few deep breaths and focus on letting all the negative thoughts you've been entertaining drain out of your body through your feet. Let the water wash them down the drain. Imagine the water landing on your head in the shower, covering you in soft white light, sinking into your skin and pushing out more of the tension, sadness, fear, anger, and even self-hatred if you harbor it. Let the steam rise around you as the water cleanses your body and energy until you can take a deep breath and feel calm.

Please note: immediately after surgery, it is likely that you won't be able to get the stitches wet. If a shower is not possible yet, run the hot water in a shower or even the sink under the mirror for a bit to create steam in the room. Add scented oil if you like it. Close your eyes, let the water run over your hands in the sink, and visualize the same white light sinking into you, pushing all the negative energy out of your hands under the water. Anoint your head or face (sprinkle some on your head and/or splash your face) with clean water flowing from the tap and know that the water itself will help that healing, calming energy sink in. It may take a little time, but you *can* cleanse this way when you don't have the strength to shower or aren't allowed one yet. When you feel calm and the mirror is foggy with steam, you can turn the tap off.

If you have a rose, a shell, or a statue of Aphrodite in the room with you, place it between yourself and the mirror. Stand in front of the foggy mirror naked and swipe a clear space in the mirror at eye level. Look into your own eyes for at least thirty seconds. Ask Aphrodite to bless you with love for the person you're looking at because they are loveable in spirit and body. Ask Her to help you accept the new way your body works, and to love the house you dwell within in this life through all its changes.

Wipe off more mirror fog, exposing more of your body. Examine the changes brought on by early treatment: stitches or scars from surgery, maybe a port in your chest for chemotherapy, even blemishes brought on by all the extra stress. Really look at them all and see that this is you surviving: this is you maintaining your spirit's house for the long haul, and the struggle leaves marks. Those marks on your body are a testament to your will to live and beautiful in their own way. This flesh is yours, and you are doing what you need to do to keep it going, to make it healthy again, and to live.

That is love. Know that She can see your love for yourself in the marks of what you've endured left behind on your skin. Take a moment to express gratitude to Her:

"Aphrodite, Goddess of Love and Beauty, I am thankful for your attention today. I will be mindful of how I think of my body. I say goodbye with gratitude."

Be sure to get dressed before the warmth of the steam fades. If you used a rose, a shell, or a statue and have the space, keep it in the bathroom near the mirror so you are reminded to look at your body with loving acceptance. Remember to close your circle and dismiss the quarters in gratitude if you've done a full ritual. Release any remaining ritual energy (and steam!) by opening a window, turning on the bathroom fan, or opening the door.

It seems like every milestone in cancer treatment brings new indignities, some endured publicly and some privately. After I recovered from surgery, I started chemo. I was weirdly grateful for being alone during some of my worst chemotherapy side effects because I hate vomiting where anyone can hear me. I feel too vulnerable and embarrassed, and I was violently ill for a few days after each of the first four infusions.

Cancer attacks your sense of dignity in so many ways and to different degrees for everyone who experiences it. I started thinking of my body as a meat-suit that was trying to kill me to distance myself from the strangers' examinations and touches. But that isn't ideal: hating your body is self-destructive, and during a critical illness it's especially important to be supportive of yourself.

Loss of dignity isn't a loss of self, and it's important to remember that this too shall pass. For better or worse, your body needs you to be gentle with it, particularly during treatment.

4

The Money

Sometime after radiation, I totaled the health insurance claims paid out for my cancer treatment. Chemotherapy is notoriously expensive: some were over $30,000 per visit. Chemo in particular is expensive because even though the drugs themselves have been around for decades, they are considered "specialty" drugs when it comes to medical and pharmacy benefit insurance. My chemo infusions were mixed in the oncology clinic specifically for me, based on my weight and prescribed cocktail. By the end of my year of surgeries, chemotherapy, labs, doctors' appointments, radiation, and a couple trips to the emergency room, I can say one of my boobs is now worth over a quarter million dollars.

If you live in a country with nationalized healthcare, this may not be an issue for you. If you're without healthcare in the US, or even if you have less-than-ideal healthcare, cancer can be a lifechanging financial burden. Deductibles, annual out-of-pocket maximums, pharmacy benefits that aren't the same as medical coverage, pre-authorizations: the financial strain of cancer and the confusing black hole of healthcare insurance can be completely overwhelming and terrifying for the whole family.

I found the social workers and care coordinators at the hospital, as well as the counselors at my oncology clinic, knowledgeable and helpful while navigating the ins and outs of medical coverage and potential financial support. In Minnesota, for example, there are local foundations that specialize in helping cancer patients pay their bills. Gilda's Club, the American Cancer Society, and Susan G. Komen Foundation all have information about financial support, and I encourage you to start with them if you're looking for resources. The websites for all three of these foundations are in the bibliography at the end of the book.

There's so much help for cancer patients because survivors and survivors' families all know how draining cancer is on the family finances. Some jobs don't have short-term or long-term disability available, stripping a cancer patient of their income—and sometimes medical coverage—when they have to stop working for treatment.

If you have any favorite money or prosperity spells, now is the time to implement them, particularly any that are repeatable over time. A few easy and repeatable money charms are below; feel free to adjust them to suit your needs.

CHARGED COINS

Materials:
- A few quarters, half-dollar, or dollar coins. Any mix is fine
- A small drawstring pouch, color and decoration of your choice

Timing:
- Full moon

Leave the coins on the pouch under the light of the full moon, preferably for the night before, the official full moon, and the night after. If you have an artistic skill to apply, it's always a good idea to embroider or draw your preferred sigil for abundance on the outside of the pouch (as easy as a $). However, that step isn't necessary if you're like me and rather artistically challenged.

After the third night, hold the coins in your hand and repeat a chant over them three times. Any chant will do if it speaks to you, such as:

> *"Coins charged by moonlight's power,
> bring abundance to my life this hour."*

Feel your own power add to the coins and pouch as you chant, adding your will to direct the Moon's magic.

Place the coins in the pouch. You can carry the pouch with you, place it on top of a stack of pending bills, or keep it on your altar as an ongoing declaration of your intentions to be secure in your finances.

ABUNDANCE ALTAR CHARM

Materials:
- A hunk of citrine (you could also use malachite, tiger's eye, or jade), for abundance
- A dollar bill
- A cleansing incense of your choice (I generally use frankincense or dragon's blood)

This can be done as part of a larger ritual or on its own. Make a space on your altar to accommodate the bill and stone (the bill can be folded). Light the cleansing incense and pass the stone(s) and money through the smoke three times. This is especially important for the money, which passes from person to person and can pick up a variety of energies on its way to you.

Hold the money in your hands. Close your eyes and visualize energy to power the spell passing from your right palm into the bill. Place the money on your altar and say:

> "I am financially secure."

Repeat the charging step with the stone(s), then place it on top of the money and state:

> "I am wealthy enough to pay my bills
> and live in comfort."

It is important to tell the universe what you want as though it's already here: that way it knows there's a gap to fill. You can leave this charm on your altar. Recharge on the days you have extra energy to spare.

MONEY CHARM

Materials:
- A green ribbon
- A dollar bill
- 3 drops patchouli oil, to attract money
- A pinch of nutmeg, to attract luck and money
- A small drawstring pouch
- Cleansing incense of your choice (such as frankincense or dragon's blood)

This charm can be created during a full ritual or on its own. Ground and center, and if you choose to cast a circle, do that now. Light the cleansing incense and pass the ribbon, money, and pouch through the smoke three times to clear the materials from external energies. Place the nutmeg in the center of the bill, add the patchouli oil, and fold it the dollar lengthwise. Then fold over the top edge of the bill to enclose the mixture.

Roll the bill up from one short end to the other and tie the ribbon around the rolled-up bill. As you place the packet in the drawstring pouch, say:

"Patchouli and nutmeg, bring money to me."

This can be combined with the charged coins or carried on its own.

As with any spell or charm, putting the energy out with the request to the universe isn't going to cut it for big, practical issues. You also have to do the work: apply for assistance, discuss your benefits with your HR person so you know exactly what your job can help with and what they can't. Reach out to your medical teams' recommendations for financial help as soon as you can, because as treatment progresses, you'll have less energy to handle the red tape involved.

I've included two long-term prosperity spells I started using before chemo began and still use today when needed. I also did the practical work of staying on top of my insurance information and support opportunities. Do your spells, do the work, keep the faith, and hang on.

SIMPLE CANDLE SPELL FOR PROSPERITY

Materials:
- Enough salt in a small bowl to stabilize a candle
- Large green candle, or any color you associate with abundance
- Matches or a lighter
- Dried basil, to invite wealth
- Toothpick, fork, or stylus

This spell works best if you can leave the candle undisturbed in a space for a period of time, because you'll be re-lighting it daily for a week or more.

Ground and center yourself, then cast your circle. It is helpful to begin this spell within a full ritual if you are inclined and able.

When you're settled and prepared, take the candle in your hands and close your eyes. Draw energy from the earth and focus on abundance: you have enough money to continue to pay your bills and live your life throughout treatment. In your mind's eye, see the energy flow up from the earth into you, and feel it rising from your feet and filling you.

Watch the abundance flowing from your hands into the candle, along with certainty that you will receive what you need to stay financially stable while you are in treatment. Take your time with this step. When your intuition says the candle is full, open your eyes and use the toothpick, fork, or stylus to carve sigils and symbols in the wax.

There is no rule here: use whatever symbols are most meaningful to you. If nothing comes to mind, it's perfectly okay to use "$." You can also carve words into the wax, if that's easier or has more power for you.

Add the dried basil to the salt in the bowl for the candle and mix gently. Create a well in the center of the basil salt and place the candle in the center. Fill in around the candle with salt to support as needed.

Light the candle while you chant three times:

"I have plenty, my bills are paid."

If you begin this spell within ritual, you may now finish the ritual and close your circle. Leave the candle burning if you can, but only if it's safe. After fifteen to thirty minutes, gently put the candle out.

Every morning for the next seven days, light the candle with your chant and allow it to burn for a time.

SIMMER POT FOR ABUNDANCE

Materials:
- Medium or large pot
- Enough water to fill the pot
- 1 medium orange, for luck and money
- 1–3 stick(s) cinnamon, for success
- 3–6 whole cloves (1–2 tsp ground cloves), for money
- A large spoon

Fill the pot to about two inches below the top and set on high heat.

Cut the orange into slices: half for a medium pot (and eat the other half), the whole orange for a large pot. Add the slices to the water and say:

"Good luck and enough money comes to me."

Add the cinnamon stick(s) to the water and say:

"A successful future comes to me."

Add the cloves to the water and say:

"The money I need to feel secure comes to me."

Stir the pot three times clockwise, and repeat the statements attracting money, success, and luck to you. Bring the pot to a boil and turn the heat down to a simmer. Let the pot simmer for as long as you like, adding water as needed (do not let the pot boil dry). Conveniently, the simmer pot smells divine and has healing and cleansing properties as well, which makes it perfect to use throughout treatment, even when energy is low.

Remember that the universe may recognize your need and assertion for abundance and money in different ways than you expected. This is a time when your friends and family will want to help with fundraisers or benefits. I've never been comfortable with that sort of help, but I realized that money is the easiest and most immediately useful way for friends and acquaintances to feel like they're offering practical support. If I had let my own pride block help the universe coordinated on my behalf, am I not negating all that magical work I'd done? I decided it's okay to accept gifts given freely out of kindness and a desire to be helpful, because maybe that's exactly how my magical work manifested.

PART II
TREATMENT

5

FACING THE LONG ROAD

My treatment plan took nearly a year, and my case was remarkably straightforward. Not easy, because nothing related to cancer is easy. The timeline of events for me started with diagnostics, followed by a lumpectomy which took two tumors out of my right breast and a couple of lymph nodes from my right armpit, then another surgery to place my chest port for infusions, then five months of chemotherapy, then a month of five-days-per-week radiation.

After radiation, I moved into what oncology calls "survivorship": six-month check-in appointments with my oncologist, daily hormone blocking pills, and a constant low-level anxiety that the next scan will be the restart of the whole process. No one is joking when they say cancer treatment is a marathon, even for those of us who have a defined timeline, and no one's treatment is identical. I know other patients who had full mastectomies right away, some who had chemotherapy for six months before surgery to shrink tumors, some lucky few who didn't have to have chemo at all. I also sat in the clinic more than once next to those who would have weekly, monthly, or even quarterly chemo sessions for the rest of their lives. Immunotherapy is becoming more popular for some cancers as an alternative to chemotherapy, but it wasn't for me. Your options are between you and your medical team, but whatever treatment plan you agree on will take time. There are no quick fixes with cancer.

My treatment began with four rounds of cyclophosphamide and doxorubicin. Doxorubicin's nickname among the nurses at Oncology is the Red Devil. I'd been warned that about two weeks after my first session of the Red Devil, my hair would start falling out. Chara, one of my oncology nurse practitioners, suggested that it may reduce the emotional trauma if I get most of it cut off before that happens. Psychologically, losing my hair becomes a choice, not something forced upon me, if I cut it voluntarily before it comes out in clumps.

I decided if this was a choice I had to make and I was headed into battle, an offering should be made. I carefully brushed my long hair and braided three individual braids, bound on either end with one black hair tie and one red. My hairdresser cut them off along with everything else, leaving me in a pixie cut with about an inch of hair so I could process the shock of baldness in stages.

I have a German Shepherd mix dog, Ragnar, who blows his coat twice per year. If you've ever had a dog with a top and undercoat, you know that during shedding season huge clumps of hair come out in your hands while you pet them, which is weirdly satisfying when you're shedding out a dog. It is less satisfying when you're shedding out your own head in clumpy handfuls. Honestly, I'm not sure it helped to process that loss in stages: if I had to do it again, I think I'd rather just buzz cut my head right away. As it happened, my sister came over when my hair started falling out and buzzed it off in a close shave, not long after she'd cut her own off in solidarity.

I kept the three braids as an offering to The Morrigan as an acknowledgement I would fight in the upcoming war knowing I would never be the same, and as a thank you for Her guidance. I've included the ritual below: feel free to use or change whatever is helpful to you.

RITUAL OFFERING OF HAIR[2]

This ritual would work well outside using a campfire or bonfire if you have the means and availability. It can be done in whatever ritual clothing feels appropriate and works with your local weather (or skyclad if you prefer), and since I tend to be as minimalist as possible with most rituals, I should say you can also do this in your everyday clothes (or pajamas, or whatever you like). I do recommend, however, taking a ritual bath or shower to cleanse and putting on clean garments that haven't been outside your space yet that day.

Materials:
- Candles: red, for Macha; black, for Badb; and white (or undyed beeswax, which can naturally be a shade from more ivory to gold), for The Morrigan.
- Matches or a lighter
- Incense: dragon's blood, for offering; frankincense, for sacred space purification; juniper berries or cedar, for healing, purification, protection; and mugwort, for healing
- An incense burner of your choice

---

[2] Please note: I used three braids for a few reasons. Three is a sacred number in many Pagan traditions. I wanted to represent past, present, and future in my offering. And, most personally, if I'd had enough hair, I would've woven nine braids to reflect the Morrigan's specific lore, but I just didn't have enough. Also, this was the last formal ritual I performed for a while, so I've included all the supplies and steps I used.

- Some amount of your own hair (does not have to be a full braid. Symbolism can be found in a small lock)
- A cauldron or fireproof bowl
- A small bowl for mixing
- 1 tablespoon Courage Oil (see recipe in Incense and Oils)
- Boline or small spoon

I begin any formal ritual by sitting or standing with my eyes closed and my hands on my knees or at my sides, and I take a few deep breaths to ground and center.

Ground and Center

Breathe in slowly and recognize any tension in your body (mine is usually in my neck and upper back). Hold that breath for a count of five to ten seconds before releasing it slowly along with the identified tension. Repeat and focus on relaxing, allowing tension to drain from your body into the earth. Become aware of your body's position in space, the places where you make physical contact with the world around you: the floor beneath your feet or knees, the feeling of your skin or clothing under your hands, any scent in the air or noise you hear. Turn your attention inward and focus on the center of your self, envisioning the light of your inner being. On an exhale, extend the light from the center of yourself deep into the earth. This can look like roots digging deep to provide a foundation of stability, or a flexible line of energy that disappears into the ground. Tension and stress flow out of you on an exhale along that line to dissipate safely in the earth, and energy flows up the cord into you on the inhale.

There are many ways to ground and center. If you've never done it, finding a way that works for you is worthwhile, because it is one of the most useful practices for treatment. It helps you stay calm, gives you an energy boost when you're exhausted, and helps you drain some of the fear and anxiety you inevitably carry along with cancer.

Light Incense

I prefer using charcoal for my incense, especially the "self-igniting" sort found at most co-op or Whole Foods-style grocery stores (and online, of course). Typically, I light the coal and set it in a container I can hold in my hands while it sparks to life. Then, I turn the container clockwise one quarter turn at a time, blowing on the coal after each turn and adding some of my own energies to the heat until the entire coal is burning.

If you use sticks or cones, note that you'll want to collect ash during this ritual, so you may need a plate or bowl as well.

Drop a small piece of frankincense on the hot charcoal. Frankincense is cleansing in both a practical and spiritual sense: there is some evidence that frankincense is antimicrobial and antibacterial as well as being an energy cleanser. There's a reason churches have used it in their standard incense blends for centuries. I know its association with Catholicism may preclude some from using it, and certainly you are welcome to substitute your preferred sacred space cleansing incense or sain instead. I use it because it's a powerful cleanser of sacred space, I wasn't raised in a church that used incense, and I'm a bit of a historian: its use is far older than Christianity. (Also, it smells amazing, which was particularly useful when many scents during treatment made me nauseous.)

After blessing yourself with some of the smoke, hold the incense burner up to each of the quarters, turning clockwise in a circle and allowing the smoke to cleanse your space.

In whatever manner suits you best, cast your circle and call the quarters. Since this book is intended for all skill levels, I've included my most oft-used wording here, but unless you're in a group ritual, calling the quarters is a very personal act. I've found that I have the same representatives of elements visiting, so I hold specific images in my mind when I'm calling because it feels like we are old friends.

After cleansing the space, before I do anything else, I stand facing north and slowly turn in place (or walk in a circle if you have the room to do so). Ground, center, and breathe deeply, drawing power up through the roots you extended into the earth. Feel that power flow through your body or into your left hand, which is at your side, facing palm down. On each long exhale, push that power out of the right hand, which is outstretched in front of your body. I usually point with my pointer and middle finger, but it's just as legitimate to use a wand, have your palm facing out, or do nothing with your hands at all. In fact, while I was sapped of all energy during chemo, I discovered closing my eyes and lying still was just as effective as walking (or turning) in a physical circle.

When you are both taking in and releasing power, visualize a pale blue light creating a circle around you as you turn, then expanding like a shield between you and the mundane world. It should fully surround you, like a protective bubble or egg (the word "circle" has always been a bit inaccurate in my opinion). As you cast your circle, say whatever invocation works best for you. I tend to say the following:

> *"I cast this circle as a sanctuary outside time and space. None may enter without my permission. As above, so below, as within, so without. The circle is closed."*

(Facing East): *"I call upon the Guardians of the Watchtower of the East, of cool air and delighted song and strong intellect. Join and protect me while I work in this circle. You are welcome here."*

(Facing South): *"I call upon the Guardians of the Watchtower of the South, of hot sand and burning fires and raging passion. Join and protect me while I work in this circle. You are welcome here."*

(Facing West): *"I call upon the Guardians of the Watchtower of the West, of deep oceans and wild emotion and hard-won wisdom. Join and protect me while I work in this circle. You are welcome here."*

(Facing North): *"I call upon the Guardians of the Watchtower of the North, of the dark forests and loamy earth and steadfast courage. Join and protect me while I work in this circle. You are welcome here."*

Light the beeswax candle. Add dragon's blood to the charcoal. Politely invite the Morrigan to the party.

Light the red candle and ask Macha for Her guidance and support in the coming battle. Add dragon's blood to the charcoal.

Light the black candle and ask Badb for Her guidance and protection in the coming battle. Add dragon's blood to the charcoal.

Add juniper or cedar to the incense burner.

Prayer to The Morrigan and Offering of Hair

1. Acknowledge that you understand this is your fight, this is your path, and though it is not a path you would've chosen for yourself, you are determined to get through it as best as possible. Appreciate that She is with you. Burn the first braid in the cauldron.
2. Acknowledge that you're scared, because only fools are unafraid before war. Promise to keep trying to not give up or give in, even though you know things will get bad. Ask Macha to lend you strength and guidance when you have no strength left. Burn the second braid.
3. Acknowledge that your old self is gone. Recognize and honor the death and loss you've experienced so far, because cancer is a death of the illusion of safety you had before diagnosis and changes the path of your life forever. Express gratitude that you have some opportunity to fight for a new life and create a new path for yourself, and that you must go through the trial of treatment as part of that transition. Burn the third braid and ask Badb for Her guidance through the transitions to come.

Add more dragon's blood, juniper or cedar, and mugwort to the incense burner (partly to cover the smell of burning hair). Meditate or pray while the braids and incense burn to ash. This is the time to sit with the Morrigan and feel Her support, express anything else you're fearful of in the coming days, or tell Her whatever else you need to say. Take time to listen for any insights or messages.

When the incense is ash, use the spoon or boline to take some of the ashes from the burner and drop them in the small mixing bowl. Add one teaspoon to one tablespoon of Courage Oil to the bowl and mix the ashes into the oil thoroughly.

Dip your index finger in the oil and draw war symbols on your forehead, cheeks, chin, across your nose—any of those spots. There is no set design here: whatever has meaning for you would be fine (including just putting a dot or line in a couple spots). I also drew symbols on my chest, particularly where I had scars, although I was *very* careful not to get any of the oil on any healing wounds, such as the stitches for my port.

When you are finished, remember to thank the Deities you've invited to the ritual for their guidance. Blow out the candles as you express gratitude and say farewell. I usually say some version of *"be welcome to stay, but if you must go, please go with my gratitude."*

Release the Guardians you've called one by one, starting with North and turning counterclockwise. Address each entity separately, thank them for their attention and protection, and release them in peace. You can use words from your own heart or start with something like:

> *"Guardian of the Watchtower of the (direction), I thank you for your guidance and protection. Please be welcome to return in peace with my deep gratitude."*

Remember to call your energies back to yourself from the circle you've cast. You can turn once more, counterclockwise, and point your left hand or just envision that blue-white light of the sphere around you returning to your body. Any excess energy can be sent back down the roots you have established for grounding, or if you feel extra tingly or overly energized, you could crouch and touch the ground with both palms for a moment. I say *"the circle is open, but never broken"* to finalize my formal ritual.

Many traditions' rituals include some version of a "cakes and wine" phase of the ceremony, whether as part of offerings to Deity or as a moment of recalling and re-grounding energy into the body. Because I was specifically offering hair in preparation for war, I did not originally include cakes and wine as part of the ritual. However, one of the reasons behind cakes and wine is to bring you back from that liminal sacred space into the real world again. I do highly recommend eating and drinking something light after a formal ritual, even if you haven't included it in the ritual itself. Ritual is a different sort of workout, expending energy while existing in a totally different space, so without a snack afterward, you could feel depleted, woozy, or a little off. I will discuss alternatives and options if you include eating and drinking as part of your practice while in treatment in a later chapter.

Ultimately, no matter what you do to empower yourself at the beginning of your treatment marathon, you'll need to constantly renew that wellspring of power through the slog of doctors' appointments, needle sticks, and sick days ahead. Resilience has you getting up the next day to try again. Courage gets you in the car to that next infusion, especially after you've had a few and know your post-chemo cycle when your anti-nausea meds run out. In the endurance test of chemo and radiation, courage gets you started, but some days it's sheer stubborn willpower that gets you through. Luckily, we witches are well practiced at honing our will to suit our purpose.

RITUAL TO QUICK-ACCESS YOUR COURAGE

Materials:
- Internet (on a device of your choice). If you don't have access via personal devices at home, most public libraries in the US have computers with free internet
- Journal or notebook
- Writing utensil
- Tiger's eye, for courage and self-confidence
- Small cloth bag (the size of a spell sachet)
- Candle and lighter or matches (not if you're in the library, of course)
    - Brown is associated with courage and grounding in that "sticking with this because it's good for me in the long run, even though it sucks now" way. However, you can use whatever color is meaningful to you for courage, resilience, and endurance. I generally use undyed beeswax candles.
    - This candle can be bigger, to be re-lit whenever you need a boost, or you can use a tea-light, small spell taper, or even a little birthday cake sized candle. If you use a smaller candle, burn it all the way down. If you use a single large one, put it out at the end of the ritual and re-light as needed.

Bring your laptop, tablet, phone, or other internet device to a quiet space where you won't be disturbed. If that happens to be your usual altar, great. If not, find a spot that will accommodate your materials and the candle.

Close your eyes and take three deep breaths. Relax your stomach muscles and let the breath expand into your core. If you're comfortable doing so, hold each breath on the inhale for three to five seconds. On the exhale, focus on relaxing your muscles and let any tension drain from your body. Repeat.

This exercise can be done with or without a full ritual. If you choose to, this is the time to cast your circle and do any of your other ritual preparations, including calling quarters and/or inviting your Deity to join.

When you're settled and centered, light the candle and place it where you can see the flame even while you're working. Then, search the internet for quotes about courage. Franklin D. Roosevelt, Winston Churchill, Maya Angelou, Cleopatra, and thousands of others have inspirational quotes about courage, resilience, and will. One of my favorites, attributed to Cleopatra, was "I will not be triumphed over." It is likely a mistranslation of the original Livy, but it worked for me the same way screaming obscenities at the toilet did when I was exhausted and miserable and empty of anything else. Rage is sometimes useful to stave off despair.

Write down anything you find that speaks to you. It doesn't matter if you have the accurate translation or the correct source; we're not going for a book report, just some inspiration. Try a few different sources, or search for people you admire, or just search for "courage." Make a list of five to ten quotes that help you access feelings of determination in the face of adversity, or inspiration that helps you stand strong against fear.

When you have your list, shut off the electronic device and set it aside. Focus your attention on the candle and meditate on the quotes you just read. Choose a favorite quote and write it on a piece of paper you can tear off and roll or fold up. Say the quote out loud as you add it to the small bag. Say it again and add the piece of tiger's eye. Close and tie the sachet and set it aside with the journal. If you've done this exercise as part of a larger ritual, complete it as you normally do and blow out the candle.

Place the candle and the journal somewhere close when you're feeling ill or low. Carry the sachet with you or keep it in your room, perhaps under a pillow, so you have a tangible example of how you want to face your treatment. Preparing for the days you won't feel strong is an act of courage and self-care.

You have the will and the perseverance to walk the road before you. Witching your way through cancer treatment is a reflection of the inner strength you have already developed. Light the candle or review the quotes that make you feel empowered whenever you need to remember that you can—and will—get through this.

6

Physical Pain and Trauma

Let's talk about the physical pain and trauma that comes with cancer, particularly with breast cancer. Whether you choose to have a partial or full mastectomy (surgically removing one or both breasts) or a lumpectomy (removing only the tumor with enough surrounding tissue to confirm the cancer is all excised), the surgeon will also take at least one lymph node from the nearest armpit to confirm whether the disease has spread to the rest of the body.

Surgery is its own sort of trauma on the body, so be kind to yourself while you recover. Use the ice packs and pain medication prescribed for recovery whenever your care team advises, because it's so much easier to stay on top of the pain than to reduce it after it's out of control. I expected some recovery pain after a major surgery, but I can tell you the absolute worst pain I felt in the biopsy and surgery process before chemo started was the radioactive tracker placed in my breast at the tumor site.

Here's where I need to put a disclaimer that this procedure is done in the US, particularly in the health system that handled my treatment. The day of surgery, I started in the same breast center where I'd had my ultrasounds and biopsies. That clinic is across a four-lane street from the hospital with the surgical center, connected via tunnel between the buildings under the street. This small architectural detail became more important than I'd anticipated.

The same team who did my biopsies handled the tracker placement in a similar process to the biopsies. I was positioned on my side on the table with my arm above my head and my breast exposed. The ultrasound tech found the tumors (at this point, a second, more aggressive tumor had been discovered through the MRI scan) and marked the spot on my skin. A new nurse, specializing in radioactive safety and responsible for tracking the tracker itself, entered with a box and a *Star Trek* style scanning tool that beeped like a disaster movie when she turned it on. She needed the beeping to prove to the doctor that the bit of metal in the box was radioactive. I did appreciate the consistency of faces: other than the fancy *Star Trek* nurse, it was the same care team who'd done both prior biopsies. First, they gave me a burning lidocaine injection, then sufficient numbing so I could watch on the ultrasound screen without any pain. Then, the doc found the tumor on the screen with the alien-needle and, instead of snapping a bite out of my body, he shot a glowing little metal tracker into my body. And that's how I became She-Hulk.

Just kidding. Truly, that would've been a much cooler outcome. But I did feel like I had some sort of alien tracking device inside. I was in a hospital gown and those purple hospital socks that have little rubber grippers on the soles. This is worth commenting on because once the tracker was in, I wasn't allowed to put my clothes back on. Instead, my belongings were loaded into a plastic bag, placed on my lap, and I was wheeled out of the clinic into the public-facing waiting room to pick up my people.

It was November 11, Armistice Day or Veteran's Day, depending on your location. Something about that symbolism seemed fitting, but I doubt there was any intent behind the surgeon's schedule. My mom and best friend came with me on surgery day, and they came along as the nurse wheeled me down to the secret tunnel under the street to the hospital with nothing on but a too-short hospital gown that wasn't fully closed in the back, weird socks, and my panties. Here's where things got uncomfortable.

About a quarter of the way through the tunnel, my lidocaine shot wore off. There is no way in hell a conspiracy theory about tracking devices shot into a person could ever work in real life, because that thing was stabbing me deep in my chest. Every time we hit a bump, I wished I could just cut it all off, because without a bra, there was nothing to support or absorb the movements.

This was one of those instances where medical staff either aren't aware it's that painful or don't mention it because there's nothing to be done about the pain. I'm telling you this now because I tend to do better with pain when I have even a glimmer of what to expect, and I went in totally unprepared.

My actual surgery and recovery were relatively easy: I'm a rule follower, so I stayed exactly on top of my medication timetables and icepacks. No ritual baths or long showers allowed during those two weeks, but none of the pain was muscular. Chemo was where the real body ache began.

The first four rounds of chemo for me were a specially-mixed-for-me cocktail of doxorubicin and cyclophosphamide. Oncology calls this combination "DC." Each cycle of DC started with my infusion on Monday afternoon, a Neulasta injection a day later, horrendous illness over the weekend, then a blood draw on the Monday after infusion for labs to check white blood cell (WBC) counts. If everything was going okay, I'd have my next infusion the following Monday afternoon, on a two-week cycle for four total infusions.

The actual chemotherapy infusion started with a nurse attaching an IV needle into the port surgically implanted under the skin in my chest. She'd take blood from the IV tube, then close it and send me back to the waiting room with the plastic tubing hanging off my chest like a lamprey eel. I'd wait for my chemo nurse to call me in and choose my chair for the rest of the afternoon, preferably one with a good side chair for my mom. The chemo chairs at my clinic were recliners with a little side table attached for holding snacks, drinks, or needles. Snacks, juice, water, and heated blankets were all offered while you hang out, which was handy since the infusions were always cold going in. The chairs had a headphone jack to let you listen to the TV. The nurse would start an IV drip of steroids and three different anti-nausea medications, which took about an hour to drip into my chest. Then I'd get the Red Devil.

Nurses and patients called it the Red Devil not because doxorubicin is one of those annoyingly long medical names, but because doxorubicin is creepily blood red in color and is the harshest of the drugs I had. While the rest of the chemo and drug cocktail could be administered by a slow IV drip while I watched TV or napped or read in the recliners at the clinic, doxorubicin came in three or four large syringes which had to be hand-pushed directly into the port IV in my chest by a nurse. The Red Devil corrodes the surrounding tissue if it drips or leaks, so there's no room for IV drip errors. It took ten to fifteen minutes to inject each syringe.

I had to get a heart test before my chemo plan was approved because my medical team needed to be sure my heart was healthy enough to handle the corrosive poison being injected almost directly into it. There is a lifetime limit on how many rounds of Red Devil a patient can have, so I live in some fear I'll have a recurrence and not be able to effectively treat any second round.

After the Red Devil, another chemo bag was hung on the IV stand (which had wheels, in case you had to pee while you're being pumped full of liquids for the afternoon). All in all, the infusion day of chemo wasn't bad, it just took a while: three to four hours each round, assuming my port wasn't clogged, which took an hour to unclog so the infusions could start.

The Red Devil kills white blood cells, which are the basis of our immune system, so while going through these first four sessions, it was vital to try to stay away from germ carriers and get my Neulasta. Neulasta is an immunity booster that works by sending the body into white-cell-production overdrive. Without it, my body couldn't reproduce white blood cells fast enough to counter the chemo killing them. At the end of each of the Red Devil infusion days, the nurses attached a Neulasta pod to either my belly or the back of my arm. The pod was about the size of a deck of cards and had a plastic injection tube that snapped into my skin like a rubber band. If the pod malfunctioned or for some reason I couldn't have it on me overnight, I would have had to go back to the oncology clinic the following day for a Neulasta injection.

The day after infusion, the pod beeped a couple times in warning and injected a drug for the next hour, putting my body into *"we must make all the white blood cells immediately"* overdrive. Neulasta was the first real time chemo caused massive pain, whether injected by the pod or in a syringe by a nurse.

White blood cells are made in the bones by the human body. The biggest bones in the body make the most cells. So, while on the drug, it felt like someone beat my upper legs, hips, lower back, and sternum with a baseball bat. And because it's bone pain, none of the usual over-the-counter pain relievers did a damn thing.

The pain lasted a couple days, and I found a hot bath with Epsom salts helped a lot. My nurses also told me to drink a lot of water for the next few days after chemo because it takes about seventy-two hours to flush it out of your system; all that water (or green tea) helps with the bone aches as well.

PAIN RELIEVING RITUAL BATH

A note on ritual baths and soaking: I was always told not to soak my port in a bath right after infusion and you can't get the Neulasta pod wet, so this is recommended for after you're able to pull the pod off and throw it away (after infusion is complete). I wouldn't lie down in even a ritual bath while I was going through chemo, because I wanted to keep my port area clean. To that end, I also avoided all public pools, steam rooms, and hot tubs while I was in active treatment (not that you'd likely have a ritual bath in any of those anyway, but seems worth mentioning).

Materials:
- Epsom salts (I like Dr. Teal's, which you can get in multiple scents, including orange, lavender, and eucalyptus)
- 20 drops (¼ tsp) arnica essential oil: from the *Arnica* plant, this oil is good for healing bruises and speeding up the healing process. Arnica is often sold in a gel for osteo-arthritis because it's anti-microbial, anti-inflammatory, boosts the immune system, and helps ease soreness.
- 10 to 20 drops lavender essential oil: use enough to give you the desired scent strength and remember it's okay to just get pre-scented bath salts. The oil is made from the lavender plant, good for relaxing the mind and body. It can be added to your bath

to calm skin irritations, relieve aches, and provide aromatherapy to help you relax. Chemo made lavender smell like soap to me, so I didn't use it as often.
- 5 to 20 (max) drops eucalyptus essential oil: Too much eucalyptus can be caustic on the skin, so be careful how much you use: not more than twenty drops in a full bath, or just get eucalyptus bath salts for convenience. It comes from the eucalyptus family of plants, good for killing bacteria and fungi, clearing sinuses, and helps the body fight respiratory infections. It also helps with arthritis so can be useful in a body-aches bath. There are a few varieties of eucalyptus essential oil available, and they all share the same benefits, but with slightly different scents. Whichever one you choose is a matter of personal preference.

Whatever scent and oil combination you decide to use, add it while the bath is running as hot as you can stand it. I like to set a relaxing mood with a candle or two and music in the bathroom, because I found all of that helped take my mind off the aches in my legs and hips. Lie in the tub, close your eyes, and breathe deeply. Just like any ritual bath, take the time to visualize healing energy seeping into you from the water, and with every exhale push a little more pain and poison out through your feet to go down the drain with the bath.

If you are a deity-minded Pagan, this is a good place to settle back in the hot water and send a prayer or chant a request for healing through a mantra or spell. If you aren't deity-minded, there's no requirement you pray or chant here. Ritual baths are a liminal space where you may have more focus and response, but if you're exhausted and just sore and sad, it's okay to just lie there and feel some relief.

I used orange-scented Epsom salts with arnica or eucalyptus; everyone reacts differently to scents while undergoing chemo, so use a combination that works best for you. The last thing you want in a ritual bath is something that makes you nauseated.

Also, if your doctor advises you to use an over-the-counter pain reliever, please follow their advice! Just because it didn't help me much doesn't mean it won't help you, and while you're going through chemo, every little bit you can do for yourself is important.

Let's talk about nausea, because my stomach has always been sensitive at the best of times and I hate vomiting more than any other illness. I'd rather have strep throat than a stomach bug. The Red Devil is a hair-destroyer and a puke-inducer. The anti-nausea drugs given during infusion wear off after a couple of days, and I was only given steroids and nausea pills through Thursday evening (by which time the chemo drugs should've been flushed from my body).

Nausea generally hit me on Saturday of the same week, and it was no joke. That first weekend, I threw up at least once per hour for about a day and a half. I still carry some trauma, physical and emotional, from the physical effects of that level of sickness. My best advice is to drink as much water as you can keep down, because dry heaving is so much worse than having something to throw up, and that level of vomiting is dehydrating. I sincerely wish for you that your experience is a cakewalk without that side effect.

After four rounds of Red Devil, I had a three week break to let my immune system recover before I started paclitaxel, or Taxol. Taxol is also a bone-ache ass-kicker and has some other unpleasant side effects, which aren't particularly painful but can be disturbing and worrisome. Taxol was originally derived from the bark of the Pacific Yew (although now it's synthesized in a lab, not harvested from the tree itself). If you're a witch with an interest in herbalism, you'll know yew, in all its incarnations, is one of the most poisonous plants on Earth. The toxin attacks nerves, which is why one of the main side effects of Taxol is neuropathy (numbness in extremities). It sounds amusing, but when your toes are numb, it's pretty easy to break them by accident or burn your fingers on the stove when you can't feel the heat level. Also, numb toes and feet can lead to clumsiness. The balls of my feet even went numb, which was disconcerting.

For me, Taxol was administered every Monday afternoon weekly for twelve weeks. As of writing this section, it's been nearly four years since I was in the throes of Taxol, and I still have occasional numbness in my middle toes and the ball of my foot.

Taxol is extremely hard on your skin, what's left of your hair, and nails. The skin on the palms of my hands and bottoms of my feet sloughed off like the aftermath of a bad sunburn a couple of weeks into my Taxol treatments. It wasn't painful but it was distressing, particularly when I reported the side effect to my oncology team because they'd not heard of that one before. I also lost the nail on my right big toe, which was also not painful at all but extremely disconcerting and worthy of a horror movie moment. In case it happens to you, it takes a year or so for that nail to grow back.

It's never fun to be a curiosity overachiever in the medical community. Chemotherapy may have a set of mostly standard side effects, but it turns out there is always room for new and weird ones, so give your medical team updates as things pop up.

Taxol is generally easier to tolerate than the Red Devil because it causes neither nausea nor deep exhaustion. But, because it's also a chemo poison, Taxol was given to me after taking quite a large dose of steroids the day before, which is supposed to help the body stave off the pain of the poison. With the first dose I didn't feel anything, but the second week, I suddenly had horrendous lower back pain that had me squirming and tearing up in my chemo chair. Taxol can cause other muscle and bone aches as well, so those ritual baths with anti-inflammatory and pain-relieving properties help. So do heating pads and, sometimes, ice packs.

Perhaps the most unexpected pain endured over the course of treatment happened about a week and a half after radiation ended. I completed my five months of chemotherapy and had a few weeks of recovery time before I started twenty days of targeted radiation. Radiation is a weird treatment process. During the first consultation, the nurse set a beanbag pillow on an exam bed and had me lie on my back, arms positioned over my head, so my head and arms made indents in the pillow. When she had me positioned the way she wanted, she used a vacuum to suck the air out of the pillow, and suddenly it was a hardened mold for my head and arms to find the same position every time I had a session. The pillow was labeled and set aside for my first treatment.

Radiation was a breeze compared to chemo. For twenty-four weekdays in June, I went to the hospital at the same time every morning, changed into a hospital gown which (of course) opened in the front, took off my jewelry, and followed the technician for the day to the radiation room. The tech grabbed my pre-formed pillow and had me lie on the medical bed under the machine. I put my arms in the pillow mold above my head, and the tech carefully opened my gown to expose only the areas that would get treatment.

Most of my journey though breast cancer had been handled by female-presenting folk (other than my surgeon) up to this point, but the radiology techs were all gender identities. It's worth noting because if modesty and who sees your nude body is an issue for you, it's okay to speak up. It takes longer to get into the correct position than anything else: after a few minutes of adjustment, the tech left the room, closing the thick, lead lined door, and the machine woke up.

The radiation machine looks like something out of a science fiction horror movie. It looms over your head and swivels in an arc above you until it's pointing at the computer-mapped correct spot(s) on your breast. Then a little arm comes out and zaps you with an invisible beam. There's a buzzing sound. It's painless.

In my case, I had to have treatment in two areas, so the machine's arm moved and did the zapping routine a second time. Then I was done: the machine retreated and quietly went dormant, the tech came in to help me up, and I changed clothes and went home. The entire process took about ten minutes. The actual radiation took about thirty seconds.

The pain factor for radiation is burns, which the doctors like to describe as skin sensitivity and potential sunburn-level topical pain. They are excellent at monitoring your skin where you get radiation—in my case, my right breast and right armpit areas—during treatment. For me, radiation was ten-minutes of prep and about thirty seconds to a minute on the bed for zapping every weekday for four weeks. It became an easy routine, and honestly, other than cumulative exhaustion that hit hard in weeks three and four, I didn't experience a lot of side effects. I'd been using lotion (both homemade and the radiologist's recommended store brands) and plain aloe gel multiple times per day, and during my zaps I had little more than a light sunburn.

Radiation burns are sneaky because they start deep inside and work their way out. About a week after I was done with treatment and ready to celebrate, I had a horrific, oozy, painful burn across the lower part of my armpit to the edge of my breast. It was so bad I could barely wear clothes, and I sobbed in the shower. The only real recommended treatment was to continue using aloe and approved lotions and take an over-the-counter pain reliever. I wish someone had told me this was coming, so I'm passing it along for you to plan. Use the softest, coolest washcloths to soothe the burn pain. If you make your own lotion, use *no* scents or essential oils, but definitely take some time to charge it with intent and energy if you have any to spare. Plan on using heavy duty sunscreen for any healed radiation burn skin for the rest of your life: I have more noticeable scars from radiation than I do from my lumpectomy, and the skin there will always be extra sensitive to sunburn.

BASIC INSTANT LOTION FOR RADIATION BURNS

Materials:
- Jojoba oil: this is the closest oil to what your body produces for your skin and hair, so it's both gentle and easy to absorb. You could also use a light carrier oil such as avocado, grapeseed, or almond, depending on your allergies and preferences.
- Pure aloe vera gel or jelly: if you have your own plant, you can use that, but it is also fine to buy aloe. Whatever aloe you use needs to be pure. Do not use the sort with lidocaine or additives that are often included for sunburn care.

Put about a dime-sized dollop of aloe vera gel in the palm of your hand. Add five to ten drops of jojoba oil. Mix with the tips of your fingers until the oil is incorporated into a white cream. Use the lotion on your face, radiation area, or other spots that need moisture and healing.

If you make more than a small dollop for instant use, keep the remainder in a small lip balm pot or jar for no more than a day or two, preferably in the fridge. This is not a shelf-stable lotion.

A note about essential oils, flowers, or herbs: if you're using something scented to augment the basic lotion, please be aware that some oils and plants which normally work great for your skin may not be good for burns. Burned skin is also very sensitive to infection, so keeping everything sterile is extremely important.

A Few Potential Additions

- **Calendula:** associated with Apollo, calendula is a powerful healing flower. Calendula is specifically listed as useful for radiation burns: it helps heal blisters and is both antiseptic and anti-inflammatory. Marigolds are a calendula, so if you can't find the petals in your local store, you can always use marigold blooms. Crush the petals and add to homemade soap or lotion. Because calendula immediately helps burns, add it to a cold compress as many times a day as needed for blister and burn relief.
- **Chamomile:** not only useful as a soporific tea, chamomile is also anti-inflammatory and antibacterial. Add to a cool compress, salve, or lotion.
- **Comfrey:** like aloe, comfrey has a high content of mucilage, which is soothing to skin. It can be added to homemade salves or lotions to promote surface healing of the skin, but because it works as a sealant, it's important to make sure the wound is meticulously clean and dried before applying any cream with comfrey added.

- **Lavender:** pure lavender essential oil is antiseptic and analgesic, which means it's soothing and helps to prevent infection. A few drops can be helpful if you have surface-level burns.
- **Witch Hazel:** witch hazel is easily found in regular grocery stores or pharmacies as well as co-ops or magical shops, usually in the facial skin care section. It's used as an astringent and reduces swelling while promoting healing. I found witch hazel too strong for any open burns, but I did use it to sooth the closed radiation burns (those that weren't weeping) before applying my salves. It can also be added to a cool compress.

In all cases of adding essential oils, herbs, or other additives to your burn care, please make sure you test on a patch of healthy skin before adding to a burn treatment. One of the common side effects of chemotherapy is resetting your histamine response, so your BC (before cancer) allergies may be significantly changed (or even gone) after chemo, and even if your favorite plants and oils worked perfectly in the past, they may induce different reactions now. I had horrendous spring and fall hay fever allergies before chemo, and for a year after treatment ended, I had no allergy symptoms at all. Slowly they've been returning, but at a reduced severity.

Whatever your side effects are during your cancer treatment, remember that it's okay to focus on yourself during this trial. Often, witches and Pagans are more in tune with their body's cycles and sensitivities, which gives you a head start at mitigating your side effects to the best possible result. But remember to be patient and gentle with your body: it's the only meat suit you get in this life, and it's working itself to exhaustion trying to stay alive for you. Feed it, rest it, and pamper it as well as you are able, because you deserve it.

Psychological Pain, Trauma, and Exhaustion

Cancer is a massive psychological trauma, full stop. Much like accounts of medieval squires going through some horrid trial to become a knight, cancer is a series of physical and mental trials that will forever change you. What (and who) matters in your life may drastically change. The journey through treatment is full of disappointments and setbacks, particularly for those who need to have some surety in their daily routine. Medical experts in the various stages of treatment are experts who have seen a lot, but the simple fact is everyone reacts differently to the stresses of cancer. And cancer is a massive stressor in every aspect of the patient's life and the lives of those closest to them: beyond the physical traumas of surgery, poison, and burning, there are the psychological, emotional, and spiritual traumas which constantly attack a person's resilience and will.

My original treatment plan didn't include chemotherapy; I was supposed to have a lumpectomy followed by radiation. Bing bang boom, I'd be done with cancer before Yule that year and be back to whatever normal looks like as soon as possible. Pathology after surgery confirmed the smaller second tumor was more aggressive, and while the surgeon was sure he'd gotten everything visible, there could still be the odd cancer cell floating around in my body. So, I was Schrödinger's time bomb: I both had a recurrence brewing and didn't, because anything that could grow into a new tumor was too small to find.

I found out I needed chemotherapy during my first meeting with my oncologist, later in the same day I'd met with my surgeon who thought everything was healing just fine. Apparently, the pathology results had come in after our appointment, so my new oncologist got the fun duty of telling me instead of wrapping this up in the next month, I'd be in for a longer battle ahead. That morning, I'd been on the quick road to recovery and moving on with my life. My surgeon and I even discussed how long I needed to heal before I could go back to martial arts classes: he expected I'd be back to mostly normal life by January.

Instead, that afternoon, the day before Thanksgiving, I found out I had five months of chemo before I could finish up with radiation, and instead of an easy fix, I would experience some of the most terrible chemo side effects. I cried for a while in my oncologist's office: this was a huge setback. It wouldn't be the last.

If you're facing the beginning of chemotherapy, you have every reason to be afraid. It's the hardest thing I've ever done; it's a miserable marathon of suck. I was incredibly lucky, which sounds ridiculous when discussing cancer, but because my cancer is extremely common (80% of breast cancer patients have hormone positive invasive ductal carcinoma, meaning my own estrogen and progesterone hormones feed the tumors) the path forward had been walked by many brave women before me. That doesn't make the path easier, it just has fewer nasty surprises and hidden traps along the way.

There's an ongoing discussion among patients and former patients about whether cancer treatment should be discussed as a war. A lot of the language we use when we talk about cancer is aggressive military language—a battle, fighting, succumbed—as though we are the three-hundred Spartans standing against a foe that could overrun us. I spent most of my treatment doing the same. I am dedicated to a goddess of conflict, death, and sorcery, after all. But there are other ways to think of treatment. Cancer treatment doesn't have to be a war with a series of battles, if that doesn't work for you. It can be a crucible in which the intensity of our will to survive and thrive is tested.

Healing is never easy on the body or mind. If you've ever broken a bone, you know the pain involved in the healing process: does the healed portion tell you when it's going to rain, even long after it was broken and fixed? Is the bone forever changed in a way that creates a new version of what feels normal, but also stronger in the place where it was broken and healed? Treatment is a whole series of awful moments which feel out of your control, but getting through them and doing the work to heal afterward will bring you to a new, potentially stronger, normal.

Have you struggled with mental illness of any kind? Have you participated in therapy or taken medications with medical guidance to help you regulate your illness? Do you consider that a battle, or just part of the journey to help you stay as healthy as possible? Shadow work, like therapy, is a whole bunch of hard, emotional, exhausting labor.

If we're honest with ourselves, healing is no picnic in any of the realms, but it doesn't have to be considered a battle. You could consider treatment as preparing the soil for the next phase of your life, particularly if you're lucky enough to have a cancer that is curable. Instead of considering it a fight, consider it a garden you're working hard to prepare for spring planting. There are possibilities coming, but clearing the way is miserable, sweaty, hard labor.

No matter what your prognosis is, *you* decide how you proceed. Witches are notoriously and gloriously strong willed because we've developed and honed our will to connect to the universe and shape our surroundings. That is vitally applicable here, regardless of cancer stage or treatment step. Whether your prognosis is a potentially full life span or a few more months, your attitude toward the time you have and what you'll do with it makes all the difference in how you deal with what comes next. I can't say what is the right treatment or path for you, but I can say I was able to ride out the worst of treatment by reminding myself that this, too, shall pass, as all things are cyclical, even the cycle of life itself.

I have always been drawn more to warrior deities. Before dedicating myself to the Morrigan, I worked most often with Artemis and Freyja, Greek and Norse goddesses of wild women and war. So, it made sense to me to aggressively evict this invader from my meat suit, because it's *my* home for this lifetime, and unwelcome intruders can get the hell out.

I am a huge fan of therapy, and I truly wish I'd found a therapist before I was in survivorship so I could've had more help during treatment. I did find a cancer mentor through a fabulous organization called The Firefly Sisterhood, a breast cancer big sister/little sister style one-on-one mentorship program in my state. I also checked out support groups through Gilda's Club (an international cancer support nonprofit named after Gilda Radner after she passed from ovarian cancer). Gilda's Club includes family and caregiver support, individual and group support, and all sorts of education and activities for cancer patients. I highly recommend them if they're in your area. Unfortunately, a good chunk of my treatment was done during the COVID-19 pandemic lockdown, so I was unable to attend groups until long after I was in therapy after active treatment was over. The following ideas and techniques I used during treatment are not intended to be done instead of professional therapeutic support, but in addition to whatever community, personal, or professional support works best for you.

LIGHT A CANDLE EVERY DAY

I don't care who you pray to, or if you pray at all. Lighting a candle every day and just focusing on the flame for a while is a reminder to your subconscious that there is still hope.

And while we're on the topic of ways to perform self-care for your psyche, try to take at least ten minutes to meditate every day. Daily meditation—with or without candles, incense, or aromatherapy—helps you develop a space between your emotions and your reactions, which gives you time to decide if a reaction is appropriate. This is especially useful if you live with others while you're going through treatment, because being exhausted and ill will make anyone snippy. Daily meditation also gives you a chance to more easily hear any messages your Deity is sending, and easier is the name of the game during treatment.

MAKE GREEN TEA OR LEMON TEA WITH A GOOD DOLLOP OF HONEY

Fluids are important when you're constantly sick, and honey will soothe your poor angry throat. If you like the flavor, green tea is a superfood with antioxidants, plus there's less caffeine than coffee or black tea. Every little bit helps. Make tea a healing spell by slowly stirring in honey, clockwise, and repeating a mantra three times, such as:

> *"I drink this cup of healing tea*
> *Help me to be cancer free."*

MEDITATE ON WAYS TO REDIRECT YOUR ANGER

In the case of cancer, anger is a powerful emotion to direct at your disease. When you don't have any other way to raise energy, it's okay to use that anger to keep going. Sometimes, sheer stubborn will and anger at the unfairness of the state we're in is the most energy we have, so why not add it to your cancer arsenal?

SPELL FOR STAYING POSITIVE WHILE THROWING UP

Gather up whatever energy you have and scream an angry and defiant *"fuck you"* into the toilet. It helps, even if you do it while crying.

FIND AND EMBRACE HUMOR WHERE YOU CAN

I don't have a specific chant or spell for this one, but I do have an inappropriate story or two. I went to the emergency room twice during chemotherapy. My mom (a retired nurse) and my care team said it'd be rare and lucky to *not* end up in the ER at least once during chemo, so two wasn't too bad.

The first time I went was after throwing up so many times I'd started throwing up blood. My sister drove me to urgent care. The mortified look on the urgent care desk nurse's face when I came in and said "hi, I'm in the middle of chemo for breast cancer and I just threw up blood" is still funny as hell when I think about it.

She said, "oh no, no, no. We don't do that here. You need to go to the ER right now. Do you need directions?" and shooed us right back out the door.

It turned out there was zero wait time for a chemo patient in the emergency room. I approached the desk nurse with the same intro and didn't even have time to sit in the waiting room: she sent me to the door, and I was immediately escorted back to a room. Was it a quiet night? I assume so, since I wasn't bleeding out or in an active heart event and I still got to a room without waiting.

A nurse helped me strip to the waist and put a gown on, and then I waited. Doctors looked down my throat and took all my vitals and asked what color the blood was and whether I'd been throwing up long. Apparently you can vomit hard enough to cause scrapes in your esophagus, which bleeds bright red (fresh). If the bleed was in my stomach, it would've been a darker color. Ultimately, it was essentially a scrape that would heal on its own, so I was offered a lidocaine/Maalox mix to settle my stomach and numb the aggravated tissue.

The nurse handed me a little clear medicine cup about the size of a Jell-O shot with a horrid, viscous, milky liquid in the bottom. I looked him in the eye and said "um, you know what this looks like, and I'm *not* a swallower. What the hell."

He barked out a surprised laugh as I slugged the potion and tried not to gag at the texture. No judgement here if that particular act is your gig, but the comment made us both laugh, and inappropriate jokes have always helped me with awkward, anxious moments. The concoction did help once I got it down, but I needed water right after, which also felt weird to drink since lidocaine is a topical analgesic and my mouth and throat were numb by then.

The best way to keep your spirits up during treatment is to find whatever humor you can. Humor is the key, and so many things are embarrassing, undignified, or plain absurd that finding even gallows humor helps.

CUDDLE

I don't care if it's your spouse, your kid(s), your friend(s), or your pet(s): cuddling on a couch or in bed while watching a movie, reading a book, or just napping does wonders for loneliness and fear. Cuddle whenever you can.

CONNECT WITH YOUR BODY

In your meditations, take time to really feel your body. I usually do this in bed before sleep and first thing in the morning because it's a good attention check-in, it gets me to start my day in as relaxed a state as possible without sleeping, and, at bedtime, it allows me to fall asleep easier. Close your eyes and focus on your breath without making any changes to it. Just observe. As your breathing naturally gets deeper, feel how it fills your lungs. Let that breath fill into your diaphragm and feel the fullness in your chest. Feel your heart beating. Unclench your jaw and let your tongue fall from the roof of your mouth. Keep breathing. Allow the muscles in your forehead to relax. Let your eyes and cheeks be soft and expressionless. On a deep breath's exhale, let your shoulders drop from where you're holding them by your ears and allow your neck to relax. Working with your breath, gently move down your body and relax as much as possible until your physical form feels heavy. If you've worked in astral projection or deep meditative journeying, this should be something you've practiced, but in this case, the goal is only to listen for any messages your body is giving you. Do you feel ill today? How is your breathing? Where do you feel pain? Itchiness? Irritation? Spots that are too cold or too hot? Cramping or other discomfort? Are you thirsty? Are you hungry? Is your nose stuffy or do you have a cough?

Once you've checked in with your body, check in with your emotional state. Are you sad today? Encouraged? Lonely? Are you starved for touch and need a cuddle? Angry? Self-pitying? Do you feel guilty for missing family, friend, or work obligations while you heal? Are you despairing? Whatever you're feeling is completely valid and you need not pile onto any negative feelings with remonstrations or additional guilt. Instead, remind yourself that this emotion will pass and sit with it until you can let it go for the time being, and do a follow-up scan of your body for any new tension that may have risen with bubbling emotions. Come out of the meditation when you're ready.

It's too easy to blame ourselves for getting cancer and to turn that blame into self-punishment. Despair lurks in closets where your clothes no longer fit the way they used to, kitchens that house food you feel sick just thinking about, bathroom mirrors that show you how much hair you've lost, or the toll chemo and radiation are taking on your skin. Despair haunts all the time during treatment and often springs while we're alone in the dark. You are 100% allowed to feel self-pity and sorrow and all the "why me" you need, but true despair will try to convince you to give up, which puts you at odds with your body's attempt to heal. If you get nothing else out of this chapter, I hope you read the next two sentences.

Please, be gentle and kind to yourself. You are doing the best you can in the situation you're in with the tools you have available, and that's all you need to do.

8

Incense, Oils, and Scents that Won't Make You Puke

Chemotherapy screws up almost everyone's senses of smell and taste. Some scents dull to the point that you may not be able to smell them at all. Some instantly induce nausea, even favorites you've used in candles, oils, potpourri, or incense for years.

    I had to stop burning almost all incense blends or smoke bundles during treatment because the smoke often gave me a massive headache or made me sick. During my Red Devil infusions, I also had to stop burning indoors entirely: I couldn't tolerate smoke regardless of the variety. Once I was done with those infusions, I could use cedar, juniper, and rosemary to cleanse rooms.

    Different chemo drugs have different effects which can also be drastically different from person to person, so the scents that are comforting without making you ill can change as your treatment cocktail changes. Through trial and (occasionally terrible) error, I discovered the following scents worked best for me during chemo, if I didn't stay in the smoke for too long.

I used dragon's blood, whether burned as incense or added to essential oil, consistently for physical and spiritual cleansing. A friend of mine considers dragon's blood to be the spiritual equivalent of bleaching, so I burned it at least once a week with the window cracked, even if I had to leave the room until the smoke cleared, because it soothed my spirits. I went through chemo during the worst months of a Minnesota winter, and dragon's blood helped keep my bedroom from feeling like an oppressive sickroom when the temperature dipped below zero so I couldn't open the window. I do recommend burning a small test batch after you've started chemo, though, even if you liked it in the past. It has a strong physical scent that hangs around after the smoke dissipates.

Frankincense is the one incense that never made me sick throughout chemo (although I couldn't tolerate the smoke during Red Devil and needed to be out of the room when I used it). A couple of years prior to getting diagnosed, I was looking for frankincense online and ordered what I thought was a two-ounce bag. It was a two-*pound* bag. Two pounds of tree resin is a lot; I had enough frankincense to run a Catholic censer for quite a while, which my witchy friends and I all found hilarious. I still have some of that bag, but I used more of it during chemo than I have before or since. I found the cleansing properties comforting and warm while dealing with the emotional and physical fallout of being so ill, and frankincense combines nicely with dragon's blood.

Eucalyptus oil helped when the Red Devil had me throwing up so often my sinuses were swollen and irritated. Over the course of the first four rounds of Red Devil, the cold I'd started with became bronchitis, and then a sinus infection. A few drops of eucalyptus oil under my pillow, in a bath, or in a diffuser helped loosen things up in my lungs and sinuses.

Lemon oil has always smelled clean and bright to me, so I used lemon often in my diffuser, particularly when I needed a boost of energy. My shampoo and conditioner have been lemon-scented or had some lemon oil added to it for years in hopes of boosting my non-morning-person energy levels before the workday. That worked until my hair fell out, but a little lemon oil on a cleaning rag or a drop or two on a bath towel, pillowcase, or even whatever you're using as a headcover helps. Lemon never made me feel ill; instead, I found it soothing when I was nauseated.

Orange oil is my other go-to for energy. It's slightly sweeter than lemon, so its scent is gentler but still motivating and energetic. Both orange and lemon are great essential oils to include when you're trying to build energy for doing anything during chemo, whether you're doing a metaphysical ritual or just trying to get the dishes washed.

Juniper oil is a scent I often mix with orange, even now. I enjoy most of the pine-y scents, but juniper was the strongest for me during chemo, so I preferred it over cedar, my go-to forest scent for many years. Juniper and orange oil mixed in a diffuser is a lovely combination.

Cinnamon, clove, ginger, and allspice, if they smell good to you, can be comforting in combination or alone. They are warm, spicy (and pumpkin spice latte) scents that also cleanse and protect. I couldn't drink coffee during chemo, but I had a little sachet of this spice blend in my linen closet to bless and pre-scent my towels.

Scent-induced nausea is one of the most known and thoroughly hated side effects of chemotherapy. Finding scents that help alleviate nausea for you is an excellent goal, regardless of the metaphysical properties of the scent. This is not the time to have your usual protection or healing scents if they make you want to throw up. It's okay to find something new, even if it's temporarily.

A note about carrier oils: chemo and radiation can make your skin particularly sensitive, far more than it is normally. I still stick to almond, grapeseed, or jojoba oil as a carrier, but everyone has different sensitivities and allergies. Please do a small test before you commit to a full bottle, and please be *so* judicious when blending essential oils with the carrier until you know how things will work.

For the entirety of treatment, I stuck to jojoba oil because I found all other oils irritated my skin. Chemo made my skin dry and extra sensitive, and the perfumes in lotions made me ill. I used plain jojoba oil or a combination of jojoba oil and aloe in a quick lotion instead of commercial products for a few months and switched to old-school Ponds cold cream during my Taxol weeks because it was extra moisturizing. If you make your own soaps and lotions, keep your sensitivities in mind: you may need to change your favorites for a time to accommodate your new normal.

I've used a couple of different oil blends over the years, mostly close to Cunningham's *Encyclopedia of Magical Herbs* correspondences, but also with my own associations over time. For the most effective infusion of energy, I generally create oil blends during a full ritual, mixing in sacred space before asking for the Morrigan's blessing. During chemo, when my energy was too low to do a ritual, I would light an unscented candle, focus on the flame, and take three deep breaths to focus my attention before I began.

COURAGE OIL BLEND

I used this blend when I needed a boost of courage, determination, or felt I was heading into battle. I've used it in rituals as well. Please note that essential oils cannot be used before surgery (in my experience, pre-op showers include a special soap that strips everything off your skin to prevent infections).

Materials:
- 1 tablespoon jojoba oil (or other preferred carrier oil)
- 3 drops dragon's blood oil, for potency, and because I often offer dragon's blood to the Morrigan
- 3 drops orange oil, for luck
- Pinch ground cinnamon, for spirituality, healing, power, protection, and success
- Pinch ground clove, for protection
- Pinch ground thyme or 5 drops thyme oil, for courage
- Small container with airtight lid (such as a small vial with a stopper)

Mix all ingredients thoroughly, save in a container with a lid, and keep out of direct sunlight. As always, if the scents, carrier oil, or herbs included in this don't work for you, change them to whatever is meaningful to you.

OIL TO COMBAT NAUSEA

Under normal circumstances, I'd use peppermint and ginger (in both oil form and ingested as tea) to combat nausea, because both are well-known stomach-settlers. Unfortunately for me, the smell and taste of both upset my stomach during chemo, so I had to find a different blend that helped. The following mix of oils worked for me instead. I used it in a diffuser more often than anything else because it worked quietly in the background while I went about my day.

Materials:
- 1 tablespoon carrier oil (if using on skin)
- 3 drops lemon oil
- 3 drops neroli oil
- 3 drops thyme oil
- A small container with airtight lid (if saving)

To use in a diffuser or a bath, add equal parts of all three essential oils to the water. You can adjust amounts for a larger volume of water, but please test it on your skin before adding extra to a bath.

OTHER OIL COMBINATIONS TO TRY

Use the same process as above to mix the following combinations as needed. All of the recipes below use one tablespoon of carrier oil and a small container or vial.

Abundance

- 9 drops yarrow oil
- Citrine or tiger's eye chip (small enough to fit in the container)

Anti-Nausea Alternative

- 9 drops peppermint oil
- Pinch of ground ginger (shake well before applying)

This recipe is better on cloth than on your skin.

Energizing

- 5 drops lemon oil
- 5 drops thyme oil

Healing

- 5 drops frankincense
- 5 drops myrrh

Peace

- 6 drops juniper or cedar oil
- 3 drops sweet orange oil

Protection

- Kitchen olive oil as the carrier
- Pinch of ground flax or 6–9 whole flax seeds
- 6–9 drops fennel oil or 6–9 fennel seeds

If you use seeds, set the sealed vial in a cool, dark place for a few weeks to a month to allow the seeds to infuse the olive oil. Use a dab for protection on your wrists as needed, or use to draw protection sigils on your doors and windows at home.

Protection Alternative

- 6 drops eucalyptus oil
- 3 drops parsley oil or pinch of dried parsley

Soothing

- 6 drops neroli or lavender oil

If you want to wear it, I found a dab of the mix in carrier oil on my collarbone or behind the jaw helpful. Put a few drops of the oils on a cloth you can carry in a pocket if you like the scent combination but your skin is too sensitive during chemo.

An easy and low-energy way to use magical scent combinations is with a room spray. There are two basic recipes for room spray, both of which I've included below along with different essential oil combinations, but please use whatever scents work best for you. It truly isn't worth using any scents that are magically beneficial but make you sick: during treatment, stick to scents that help you soothe symptoms, cleanse sickroom miasma, or affect your energy levels (whether that's helping you sleep or pumping your energy up).

BASE ROOM SPRAY ONE

Materials:
- Small funnel
- 4 oz spray bottle
- ½ teaspoon vegetable glycerin (often found in organic section at the grocery store, or in co-ops or Whole Foods stores)
- 25–30 drops of essential oils (total)
- Distilled water to fill remainder of bottle

BASE ROOM SPRAY TWO

Materials:
- Small funnel
- 4 oz spray bottle
- 25–30 drops of essential oils (total)
- Witch hazel (equal parts to water)
- Distilled water (equal parts to witch hazel)

When it comes to essential oils for room sprays, any of the combinations in the Oils section would work. However, it's important to note that the room spray may have a more powerful scent, acting more like a room diffuser than a dab on the wrist. Stick to your favorite helpful variations.

Soothing/Relaxing

This can be adjusted to your particular scent tolerances by increasing one or the other scent. Whichever you increase should be offset by decreasing the other (twenty drops of cedar would mean reducing lavender to ten, for example).

- 15 drops cedar oil
- 15 drops lavender oil

Energizing and Mood Boosting

- 15 drops grapefruit, lemon, or orange oil
- 5–10 drops eucalyptus oil
- 5–10 drops tea tree oil

Note: grapefruit oil may suppress appetite, which is not what you may need during treatment. However, it is an antibacterial and antimicrobial mood-booster, so I use it in the bathroom. Lemon or orange oil also helps boost mood and can be used with the other oils in this recipe based on your own preferences.

Love

- 15 drops sandalwood oil
- 10 drops vanilla extract

Magical and Physical Cleansing and Protection

- 10 drops rosemary oil
- 10 drops thyme oil
- 10 drops frankincense oil

Clarity

- 5 drops basil oil
- 10 drops lemon oil
- 10 drops rosemary oil

You could swap grapefruit or ylang-ylang for lemon, although please note my comment above on grapefruit's appetite suppression, and be careful with (or enjoy) ylang-ylang, as it can have an aphrodisiac effect. Peppermint could also be added or substituted for rosemary. Like all your fragrance decisions, the mix depends on what your treatment tolerates.

You may have noted my use of traditionally flowery scents in the above combinations is sparing. During chemo and radiation, I either couldn't smell most flowery scents at all, or they made me terribly sick. Gardenia, honeysuckle, rose, and other flower essences have their own lovely effects, and I encourage you to substitute where appropriate. I just can't recommend those combinations because I couldn't use them. Test and retest what works best for you during your treatment, because your tolerances and preferences can change with every new infusion.

9

Magical Eating

Cancer is hell on your entire digestive system. Stress, post-op painkillers, chemo infusions, side-effect management drugs, and radiation all take a heavy toll that suppresses your appetite, even though you need energy to heal. Foods taste like paste because the drugs deaden taste buds. Nausea, vomiting, sore throat and esophagus, and diarrhea are common side effects, so even though healthy foods like vegetables, salads, and lean protein are ideal, they aren't always easy to handle. Mouth sores can happen, which reduce food options even further, since anything with citric acid or capsaicin will just burn. It's exhausting and disheartening, particularly if you're a foodie. I had cheesy mashed potatoes for a week straight once because it was soft, easily digestible, and mild if I couldn't keep it down.

Eating while you're going through treatment is tricky, because your body needs nutrients to heal, but it's often difficult to eat anything. If you're in treatment now, your health care team should be working with you on your nutritional needs and how to meet them. This section is not intended to replace your medical resources, but to give you some ideas and options I used and maybe inspire you to add a spice or herb here and there that can magically assist. I felt much perkier on the bad days when I had soft scrambled eggs, hummus, or yogurt to provide a good amount of protein, which is useful to the body for healing and rebuilding immunity.

The following list isn't exhaustive at all: part of your healing includes figuring out what works for you both magically and mundanely. If you don't happen to have something in your cupboard already, don't stress about rushing out and buying new spices. Chemo changes the flavor of our favorite foods so drastically it's possible something you love will be awful, and something you learn to love while in treatment will be awful after it's over. The following list is the food, herbs, and spices I was able to eat or smell without getting sick so you have a place to start.

A disclaimer: please check with your medical team often to be sure the herbs and spices you're using don't interact badly or interfere with your medications.

ALLSPICE

Allspice magically promotes healing via ingestion or aromatherapy. Include it in baking, soups, tea, ritual baths, sachets, and other scent-centered endeavors. Allspice smells wonderful and can be combined with other spices such as cardamom, cinnamon, cloves, ginger, or nutmeg.

ANISE

Anise seed and star anise have strong licorice-like flavor. Used in cooking, it's aromatic and slightly sweet, so it's especially great for baked goods. It can be combined with other common spices for tea, ritual baths, and sachets. Anise and bay in conjunction is a powerful form of purification, and anise can be used when calling spirits for assistance and protection.

APPLE

Used in love spells, spells for the dead, healing spells, and as a symbol of immortality, apples are a magical superfood. *Illustrated Herbiary* by Maia Toll has a lovely ritual with apples to discover and accept your whole self, even the hidden parts. She says: "The self begins in our physical body and everything it can feel, taste, see, hear and smell." (Toll, 34) Focusing on observing all your senses while eating an apple is particularly useful when cancer makes you feel like your body is no longer your own. Apples are easily digested (particularly without the peel) and can be combined with other magical spices, such as cinnamon or nutmeg, to be a sweet, edible healing spell. Apples are listed on the AICR (American Institute for Cancer Research) cancer-prevention diet.

BANANA

Bananas are an excellent source of energy in a smoothie or on a bad-guts day because they're soft and bland. Magically, bananas are used for fertility and prosperity spells. Let's be honest: cancer is a bitch on the wallet in any healthcare system, so if you're in need of some monetary help, cook up some delicious banana bread and infuse the batter with intent to draw prosperity to you while you stir (clockwise, of course).

BARLEY

Magically, barley provides protection and healing. One of the spells in Cunningham's *Encyclopedia of Magical Herbs* says to wind barley stalks around a stone, visualize your pain going into the stone, and toss it into running water to wash it away. (Cunningham, 47) It's probably not the most practical spell if you don't have barley stalks, but if you like barley in your soup, why not use that sticky magical quality? Visualize the barley pulling sickness out on its way through your body and flushing it away. Nutritionally, barley is a complex carbohydrate and it's gentle on a sick belly, so adding to soup is useful and tasty.

BASIL

Included in the list of herbs that reduce free radicals, which are the compounds which promote abnormal growth in breast cancer patients among other damaging bits of nastiness. From a magical standpoint, basil is primarily used for love spells, exorcism, protection, wealth, and, apparently, flying. I wasn't flying while I was on chemo, but it could be useful for wealth and protection spells. It also still tasted like basil while I was on medication, which helped make buttered noodles less bland.

BAY LEAF

I've included bay here for a few reasons. First, it's easy to add bay to soup or stews (pull the leaves out and discard before eating the soup) for additional flavor. Second, from a magical perspective, bay leaves have many uses for someone in treatment. One of the simplest low-energy spells is to write something on a bay leaf and burn it, sending the spell to the gods. Bay is one of the oldest herbs consistently used in magic and is reputed to have healing qualities, preventing illness just by being planted near the house, so keep some bay leaves in your kitchen and hang a sachet of them from the showerhead (or place in a bath) to imbue strength and purification.

BLACKBERRY

Berries of all sorts are considered an excellent nutritional package in general because they're full of antioxidants.

Blackberries are also potent magical healers, so I incorporated them whenever possible. They are flavorful in smoothies or yogurt if you're having issues with their texture.

BLUEBERRY

Blueberries are on the AICR list of anti-cancer superfoods and should be incorporated into your diet if you can. They still had strong flavor while doing chemo. I usually put mine in my oatmeal in the morning instead of any added sugar (since the same nutritionists who recommend these superfoods also recommend reducing your sugar intake), but who would dare tell you blueberry pie isn't magical?

CARAWAY

If you like rye flavor, caraway seeds are strong when chewed. I like rye, so I liked the occasional caraway rye bread during treatment. Magically, caraway seeds are lust and fidelity enhancers, but they're also helpful for memory and health. "Chemo brain" is a real phenomenon, where your cognition and recall may not be as fast as usual. You could include caraway in a spell sachet or include caraway rye as part of your spell if you're having memory issues.

CARDAMOM/CARDAMON

Magically, cardamom is related to love and lust spells, so I didn't use it at all for magical purposes. It smells divine, however, and adds a warm hearth-and-home quality to teas and baked goods.

CHAMOMILE

I've included chamomile here because you can get chamomile tea in nearly every grocery store in the US. It's a soporific, so it's helpful if you have insomnia. It's less helpful to drink if you're prone to hay fever allergies (like I am), but it has a lovely, relaxing scent. Add a chamomile tea bag to a pot of boiling water on the stove, or to your bath, for a calming ambiance before bedtime.

CHERRY

Cherries are on the list of superfoods my oncologist gave me to try to incorporate into my diet. They're high in natural sugar, so they give you fast and easy energy when you're exhausted. They're also high in antioxidants and have a strong, tart flavor. Cherry isn't something I used magically during treatment, though, as its magical correspondences mostly focus on love and lust.

CHILI

Whether used as a fresh pepper or dried spice, chilis can add a ton of flavor to foods during chemo. Magically, they're mostly associated with love and breaking hexes, but nutritionally, fresh chilis are a good source of vitamin C. A word of warning: use sparingly until you know if the scent, flavor, and heat will work for you. I waited on anything with chilis or chili powder until I was on Taxol because it was too strong for my stomach during the Red Devil.

CINNAMON

I put cinnamon in my tea, oatmeal, applesauce, and baking as often as possible before and after chemo. It didn't change taste during treatment at all, which was a blessing. Cinnamon is a powerful spice and oil with a wide range of uses. Include cinnamon in your incense for its healing and protective properties, use in tea or bath sachets for the same reason, ingest it to draw money to you, and offer it to your Deity.

CLOVES

From a magical perspective, cloves draw money and prosperity, protect the user from negative forces, and purify. I include cloves wherever I use cinnamon, particularly in tea and baking. My favorite blend when I have a head cold or sinus issue is black tea (English or Irish Breakfast, usually) brewed strong with a couple of teaspoons of Tang, a generous amount of cinnamon, cloves, and a dash of nutmeg, and sometimes ginger as well for a decongestant. Don't judge me on the Tang: I have a terrible addiction to sugar. A dash of orange juice would also work.

CORIANDER

If you didn't know it, coriander is also called cilantro (often in grocery stores, you see coriander describing the seeds in the spice aisle, while cilantro is the leafy herb in the produce section). Coriander is a magically healing herb: you can use the spices in sachets and spells or use them in spice blends. The green herb is delicious in salads, chili, and avocado toast, if you aren't one of the people who taste soap when chewing it. Cilantro seems to be a binary herb in that sense.

CRANBERRY

Listed in the AICR's anti-cancer foods, cranberries are tart and full of vitamin C. They are acidic, so if you have mouth sores or an irritated stomach, throat, or esophagus, you may want to avoid them, but otherwise they're an excellent flavor during treatment.

CUCUMBER

Cukes were an easily digested vegetable when I was in treatment, although, to be honest, I couldn't taste them at the time. Cucumber tomato salad gave me fresh vegetable nutrients with some crunch, and adding basil made it magically and mundanely healthy. Magically, cucumbers are used for healing, fertility, and chastity (which seems a bit incongruous, but that's magic for you).

CUMIN

Another spice I used for its strong flavor, not for its magical properties, cumin is in a lot of Mexican and Tex-Mex food. It goes well with cilantro and beans, both of which are healing foods, and it's great in scrambled eggs.

DILL

For the entirety of chemotherapy, I was unable to eat dill—including pickles—because it made me nauseated. Magically, dill is primarily for lust and love, money, and protection, so between those uses and its strong flavor, it's worth mentioning if you can tolerate it.

ELDERBERRY

Like many berries, elderberry is a healthy boost to your immune system. Elderberry syrup is now available in grocery and big box stores as a general cough syrup. The plant is also used in magic for its healing properties, from teas to tinctures to wine. When your immunity is low, try an elderberry gummy (if okayed by your doctor): hold it in your left palm, cover with your right, and take a moment to focus on healing before eating.

EUCALYPTUS

Used for healing colds and congestion since it was discovered by humans, eucalyptus is a magically healing herb as well. Hang a bunch of eucalyptus leaves from your showerhead or add some to your bath (or use the essential oil) to help clear the sinuses and promote healing. Eucalyptus has a strong astringent scent, so if it doesn't upset your stomach, it helps clear the sickroom of any lingering unpleasant aromas.

FENNEL

A truly versatile herb, fennel bulbs, leaves, or seeds can be cooked into a wide variety of dishes. Like anise, fennel has a licorice flavor which is different depending on the part of the plant. It's used for purification and healing in magic, so include the seeds in any spell mixtures for healing.

FLAX

Flax seeds are on the AICR list of foods which prevent cancer. For ingestion, flax seeds should be ground (they last longer without going rancid if you buy whole seeds to grind at home, but ground flax is often in the organic section at the grocery). I add my flax to oatmeal for the nutritional value, because the flavor is so mild it disappears when mixed with something else. Magically, flax is a healing seed to add to any healing spells or sachets: "Sprinkle the altar with flax seed while performing healing rituals or include it in healing mixtures." (Cunningham, 118)

GARLIC

Never mind vampires, garlic is a triple threat for cancer. It's on the AICR list, it's powerful flavor and scent busts through chemo, and it's a magical healing herb. Garlic is strong enough, though, that it may cause nausea. If it doesn't, use it liberally in your food to ingest the protective magics garlic carries, as well as the nutritional value.

GINGER

Magically, ginger is a heat-generator used most often in love and lust spells. But that heat and energy-raising power is useful for healing, too. Add ginger to your tea to help settle your stomach if you're nauseated, and add it to baking for extra flavor. Ginger is spicy when it's raw, so be gentle with your mouth and throat if you get sores during chemo.

GRAPESEED EXTRACT/OIL

Included in the list of herbs that reduce free radicals in breast cancer patients, grapeseed is high in antioxidants and considered anti-inflammatory. It's also high in vitamin E, which makes it a great carrier oil for lotions, massage, or essential oil blends. Grapeseed oil can be used in cooking as an alternative to olive oil or vegetable oil. Please note: the smoke point of grapeseed oil is slightly higher than olive oil.

GREEN TEA

All tea is on the anti-cancer foods list to incorporate into a diet, but green tea has a specific reputation for being a healing agent and cancer fighter. According to *Science Connected Magazine*, one of green tea's specific antioxidants, epigallocatechin gallate (EGCG), has been studied for the way it protects one of the anti-cancer proteins. The protein repairs damage on a cellular level, so EGCG acts like a bodyguard and cancer repair unit. Yes, I'm absolutely imagining tiny green sci-fi warriors watching over field engineers doing their cellular repairs, and I'm tickled at the thought. Green tea can taste a little grassy, but add a little lemon and ginger to brighten the flavor or add honey for a sore throat and drink a few cups per day.

HONEY

Honey is antibacterial and soothing if you have a sore throat or mouth sores. Its sweetness was flavorful during chemo, so I used it often in tea or on peanut butter toast.

HOPS

Alcohol (of all kinds) is on the list of things to eat less of or eliminate for cancer prevention. However, hops flowers or pods can be included in healing incense or spells. Honestly, beer tasted awful to me during treatment, but if it's your thing I'm not going to say you can't drink it. Check with your doctors, and if you do imbibe, think about the healing power of hops.

LEGUMES

Legumes include beans (kidney, navy, and the others), lentils, peas, and peanuts. They're all on the anti-cancer foods list, and they are packed with protein and fiber. Chemo made legumes taste like paste, but they are perfect vehicles for many of the spices listed here to give them a blast of flavor. Legumes are also gentler on your digestive system than meat and are soft when cooked, which makes them a perfect source of protein when you're struggling with side effects. See my recipe for magic-infused lentil soup at the end of this chapter for one way to cook with them.

LEMON

Lemon is a purifier. Its scent says "clean" to the subconscious, which makes lemon a versatile cleanser in purification spells or sachets. Add lemon to your water (hot or cold) for an immunity booster, as it's high in vitamin C, and to aid in digestion. Consider adding lemon and ginger together to your water or tea if you can tolerate it, because the combination is soothing to upset stomachs and flavorful. Lemon is also anti-fungal and anti-bacterial. Because it's acidic, it may be better for room cleansing than eating if your side effects include mouth sores.

LEMON BALM

Lemon balm makes a lovely, light tasting tea. Combined with honey, lemon balm tea is soothing for a sore throat. Since it doesn't have the harsh acidity of lemon, lemon balm is a nice flavor substitute if mouth sores or a sensitivity to acidic foods is an issue during treatment. For magical healing in non-ingested ways, add it to incense, spell sachets, or baths.

LIME

Like lemon, lime has a strong citrus tartness that cuts through deadened taste buds, so it's a great flavor to add to food during chemo. Its scent is slightly sweeter than lemon, and it's equally anti-fungal and antibacterial, so you could use it in all the same ways as lemon if you prefer the taste and scent. Also, like lemon, limes can sting and be too harsh on mouth, throat, or esophagus sores.

MESQUITE

Mesquite is most often used in barbeque or smoking meats, but it is a powerful magical healer. Include it in incense if you like the scent and in marinades for meat if you like the flavor. It's a strong flavor, so it works well during chemo, but avoid if either the flavor or scent makes you queasy.

MINT (INCLUDING PEPPERMINT AND SPEARMINT)

Mint is excellent for cancer patients. It's both mundanely and magically healing and soothing, so use liberally. Mint can help with nausea, and its flavor and scent are powerful for dampened senses. Use it in tea, baking, aromatherapy, and sachets. A few drops of mint oil in a bath are soothing, and hanging a sprig of mint leaves in your shower works similarly to eucalyptus for a refreshing, awakening experience.

NETTLE

Nettle tea is full of antioxidants, which are excellent cancer fighters. Magically, nettles are useful for protection and healing.

NUTMEG

Add nutmeg to baking or teas for luck and to promote health. Nutmeg has a subtle flavor, so it works well with cinnamon and cloves but can be lost during chemotherapy. During chemo, I included it in my usual recipes more for the magical properties than the taste.

OATS

The magical aspects of oats lean more toward prosperity and money than health, but oats (particularly in the form of oatmeal) are soothing in an upset belly and pack a good amount of nutrients in a soft, easily digestible form. They are considered cancer-fighters if they're whole grains (steel cut oats rather than instant oatmeal). Oatmeal is a carrier for both sweet and savory ingredients, so there are a variety of healthy options to try. Oats are also wonderful in a bath, as they have skin soothing and softening properties. Include them in a cloth bag or grind them into a powder and add directly to the tub for a ritual bath (or a regular one).

OLIVE

Olives and olive oil have been used for ritual, healing, and nutrition for thousands of years. Olive oil is a healthy fat to use for cooking or salad dressing. If you get extra virgin olive oil, the flavor is very light and barely there, particularly while going through chemo. Green or Kalamata olives are both salty and sour, which means you can taste them during treatment. Olive branches bring luck and encourage victory, both useful magically while fighting cancer. Versatile and nutritious, olives are a handy tool to keep in your kitchen during cancer and after.

ONION

Onion is a healing food both magically and physically, and it's a flavor enhancer. If it doesn't cause nausea, use it wherever you can in cooking to ingest both the nutritional value and magical healing properties.

ORANGE

Oranges are on the anti-cancer food list. They're packed with vitamin C, which helps boost your immune system, and while I was on an iron supplement, my doctor advised me to drink orange juice with it because vitamin C helps the body absorb more iron. Oranges were one of the things that tasted completely normal during chemotherapy. As with any citrus or peppers, if you have mouth sores or acid reflux, you may want to avoid eating them. However, the scent of orange in the home is both cleansing and gently invigorating, so include orange peel in sachets or potpourri. Orange oil is also lovely in a bath or diffuser. Magically, oranges attract luck, and who doesn't need some good luck while in treatment?

PAPAYA

Papaya brings magical protection and is a digestive aid. The seeds are poisonous, but the fruit has an enzyme that assists the body in breaking down food, so it's useful for indigestion.

PARSLEY

From a culinary perspective, this herb is mild enough that you may not be able to taste it. But magically, parsley can be used for protection and purification, so it can be eaten or included in a purification bath.

PEPPER

Black pepper can be included in sachets and spells for protection. Pepper is often dismissed as a spice because it's in every kitchen, but it is strong and can be tasted during chemo. Its major compound, piperine, increases the body's ability to use other important foods, both nutritionally and magically, including magnesium, iron, and turmeric.

PLANTAIN

Plantain magically promotes healing by drawing out illness that's sticking inside you. Plantain chips were a tasty alternative to potato chips or crackers when I was nauseated and are easily found in grocery stores. If you can find (or have the energy to make) them, mashed plantains have a similar consistency to mashed potatoes and are a bland, easily digested source of nutrition on bad side effect days.

POMEGRANATE

Pomegranates are an antioxidant-rich fruit that are associated with Persephone. I gave them in offering to Her, particularly at Yule, as a symbol of my descent into the underworld during treatment and eventual return to the light. Magically, pomegranates protect against evil. Physically, they are tart like cherries and can be tasted despite chemo. I drank the juice instead of eating the pips during treatment because the pips upset my stomach.

POTATO

The starchy wonder of potatoes cannot be overlooked in a diet for those going through chemotherapy. Potatoes are versatile, gentle, and can be a full meal just by adding some toppings. A baked potato topped with bean chili (preferably with chili powder, cumin, and cilantro), some cheddar cheese, and maybe a little sour cream is a meal packed with flavor, nutrition, and healing magic. On the other hand, when you've been vomiting up everything you ate for a few days and your insides are irritated and sore, potatoes are a bland and easily digested first step back to solid food. Magically, potatoes have healing qualities too, so, as Samwise Gamgee would say, "boil 'em, mash 'em, stick 'em in a stew" whenever you like. (Jackson, *Lord of the Rings: The Two Towers*)

ROSEMARY

Rosemary is included in the list of herbs that reduce free radicals in breast cancer patients. Its strong scent and flavor breaks through the chemo-dulled senses. Rosemary is associated with memory, so be mindful of what memories it brings up and what memories it can create during treatment. Burn rosemary in incense or a smudging bundle for magical healing and include it in ritual baths for purification, a sachet under your pillow with thyme for sleeping, or in your healing spells.

SAFFRON

Saffron is quite expensive in the US, and its delicious flavor is subtle, which are both reasons not to use it during chemotherapy. However, saffron has a reputation for helping with stomach ailments and stimulating appetite, which makes it worth a try. According to Ilana Sobo of *The Alchemist's Kitchen*, saffron was used to treat a myriad of ailments by many ancient cultures, particularly the ancient Persians, Greeks, and Romans. It has historically been used in love spells and devotional offerings to deities, and to treat melancholy (depression), so it is useful for magical and spiritual healing as well the physical benefits.

SAGE

Sage is included in the list of herbs that reduce free radicals in breast cancer patients. Magically, sage is associated with protection, immortality, and, of course, purification of ritual space. Please note white sage is endangered due to recent overcultivation and considered appropriative to use by Indigenous people who use it in closed practices, unless it's been gifted to you. However, there's no reason you can't burn regular garden sage to cleanse your space, because all sage helps clear the bits and bobs of psychic garbage that's attached itself to you or your surroundings. If you do decide to use it as smoke, be sure you declare an intent as you are burning it, because some say sage is an attention-grabber for spirits (therefore, you'll want to let them know you're clearing old junk out and that's all). Sage doesn't have a strong flavor, so you likely won't be able to taste it during treatment, but since it's both magically and mundanely useful, you may want to include it in your cancer diet and workings.

TEA

All tea is included in the AICN's list of cancer prevention foods due to its antioxidant properties. Black tea's magical properties include increasing riches, courage, and strength, all of which are needed during cancer treatment. Of course, drinking tea is the most common way to incorporate its qualities into your life, but you can also add tea leaves to a talisman for courage.

THYME

"Thyme kills off what's 'other' whether that's germs and microbes or thoughts and feelings. This is Thyme's special magic." (Toll, 45) Burn thyme in your incense to attract good health. Add it to salads, chicken, fish, and beef for excellent flavor, and add to your spells for healing. I also really liked the scent of thyme and rosemary while I was on chemo: not only could I smell them, but they also smelled clean and refreshing and, most importantly, didn't make me queasy.

TOMATO

Tomatoes are on the anti-cancer diet list for their antioxidant and anti-inflammatory traits, and they're versatile in both flavor and use. Even those who hate raw or cooked tomatoes often like them as pizza sauce or pasta sauce, as an example, and how easy is it to make magically healing sauce with herbs like garlic and basil added to the tomatoes? Tomatoes also attract prosperity to the home and offer protection. They are acidic, so wait until you don't have any mouth sores, nausea, or heartburn from treatment before eating them.

TURMERIC

Magically, turmeric is used primarily for purification. Mundanely, turmeric has anti-inflammatory qualities, and its scent is pleasant when added to food. I couldn't taste it, but I'd add to rice and noodle dishes, chicken, and chili because I could still smell it.

WALNUT

Walnuts are on the AICN's list of cancer preventing foods. Magically, they're used for health, both through ingestion and inclusion in spell work. Remember that oatmeal/blueberries/flaxseed mixture I mentioned earlier? I always add walnuts to that combo if I have them on hand for a dose of healthy fats. And, in the spirit of correspondences, walnuts look like brains—they are excellent for brain health and chemo brain!

WINTERGREEN

Like others in the mint family, wintergreen is useful during treatment in many ways. It helps to soothe an upset stomach and cleans your mouth when chewed. It can be included in teas, both the sort you drink and the sort you put in a bath, for healing. Add some leaves to your healing sachets or keep a few near you on your sicker days to have a fresh scent that clears your head and helps with headaches.

YEW

Yew is a powerful poison and should never be ingested. It's included in this list not because I used it when I was going through treatment, but because paclitaxel (Taxol) is derived from yew, so it was used on me as part of a chemotherapy drug. Interestingly, according to Cunningham, yew was "sometimes used in spells to raise the spirits of the dead" (Cunningham, 265). Boy oh boy, that seems like an appropriate magical use for chemotherapy, doesn't it? So, if you get Taxol as part of your treatment for cancer, think about how it comes from a plant that is used to raise the dead, and maybe take heart at that thought, because it's getting used medically to kill cancer and keep you alive.

FOODS RECOMMENDED BY ONCOLOGY:

- Apples
- Asparagus
- Blueberries
- Broccoli and Cruciferous Vegetables
- Brussels Sprouts
- Carrots
- Cauliflower
- Cherries
- Coffee
- Cranberries
- Flaxseed
- Garlic
- Grapefruit
- Grapes
- Kale
- Oranges
- Dry Beans, Peas, and Lentils
- Raspberries
- Soy
- Spinach
- Squash (Winter)
- Strawberries
- Tea (Green especially, but all tea is included)
- Tomatoes
- Walnuts
- Whole Grains

Based on those lists, it absolutely seems like the ideal diet is vegetarian, right? The power of healthy eating is important, but I want to remind you that while you're in active treatment, it's more important to find something you can taste and keep down. I regularly craved Burger King Whoppers (with cheese, of course) while I was getting chemo, because it was something I could taste that had protein and veggies. Was it the healthiest option? No. Did I lose forty pounds from being sick while getting chemo, so at some point, just eating anything that stayed down was the goal? Yes.

Now that I'm post-treatment, my goal is to eat as healthily as possible, basing my diet around fruits, vegetables, and legumes and considering animal protein as a side dish. There are cookbooks and websites focused on cancer prevention diets and recipes, but I will end this chapter with a few recipes I used during treatment and survivorship.

PROSPERITY PANCAKES

Pancakes are soft and easy to digest during the bad days of chemo and can be magically and practically pumped up to accommodate prosperity, health, and protection with just a few additions. Use buckwheat pancakes for extra fiber, as well as attracting money and protection. Feel free to adjust where I use dairy if you are dairy-free or vegan.

Materials:
- Cast iron pan (if possible), griddle, or large nonstick pan
- Mixing bowl
- Buckwheat pancake mix, for money and protection
- Water
- ½ teaspoon cloves (ground), for money and protection
- ½ teaspoon cinnamon (ground), for success, healing, and protection
- ¼ teaspoon ginger (ground), for money and success
- Butter

- ¼ cup pecans, chopped (optional), for money
- Any combination of the following:
  - Cashew or almond butter, for money and prosperity
  - Blueberries or blueberry jam or syrup, for protection
  - Blackberries or blackberry jam or syrup, for healing, money, and protection
  - Peaches (fresh or from a can), for longevity

Ground and center before you begin and consider your intentions for this meal: to increase your health, protect you, and attract money or prosperity.

Set the pan or griddle to medium-high heat. If you're anemic or become anemic during treatment, try to cook as much as you can in cast iron (every little bit helps), but ultimately use whatever works best for you.

In the bowl, mix the buckwheat pancake mix according to the instructions (you should only need water) with a fork or whisk. As you stir clockwise, say *"health, wealth, protection"* three times.

Add spices one at a time. Name them as you add them to the batter and say what they'll bring to you.

"Cloves, protect me."

Stir the batter clockwise once.

"Cinnamon, protect and heal me."

Stir the batter clockwise once.

"Ginger, bring money and financial success to me."

Stir the batter clockwise once. Add pecans if you include them. Repeat the process you used for spices.

"Pecans, bring me financial abundance."

Stir the batter clockwise once.

Use the butter to grease the griddle where you will place pancakes. I usually use a stick with the paper still on one half, so I can make a series of circles on the pan/griddle with the unwrapped end. Pour the pancake batter and watch them cook; you may have to adjust the temperature up or down.

If you want berries in your pancakes, add them before the pancakes are cooked through and before you flip them. Flip the cakes when the edges look dry and there are bubbles popping on the top.

op the finished pancakes with your preference of toppings. Cashew or almond butter adds protein to the pancakes. Blueberries and blackberries in or on the pancakes add prosperity. Peaches add longevity. Whatever choices you make for your preferred flavor, add your toppings mindfully, with intentions. Take your time eating and taste the unique combination of flavors you've added. Know you are ingesting luck, health, protection, and prosperity with this meal.

FORTIFYING LENTIL SOUP

Lentils are a great vegan protein with a ton of fiber that are easily digested and soft after cooking. This lentil soup recipe is easily tweaked to taste and can be made vegan by changing the broth from chicken to vegetable. Use fresh or dried herbs, just check their potency so you can taste them.

When cooking dried lentils, it's a good idea to dump them into a sheet pan and check for any accidental pebbles that were included. Then, rinse them off in a colander and they're ready to go (no overnight soaking required).

Materials (scale up or down as needed):
- Dutch oven (or any stock pot or large noodle pot)
- 4 cups chicken broth (use vegetable broth to make this vegan)
- 2–3 carrots, chopped
- 2–3 celery stalks, chopped
- 1 bunch of kale, Swiss chard, or other hearty leafy green
- 2–4 bay leaves
- 2 tablespoons olive oil
- 1 medium onion, chopped (I use red or white, not sweet yellow)
- 1 bag dried lentils (about 2 cups) rinsed and sorted, any color
- Rosemary
- Thyme
- Oregano
- Salt
- Pepper

Pour the olive oil in the pot and set heat to medium-high. Add chopped celery, carrots, and onion. Sauté, stirring regularly, until onions are clear and vegetables soften, about ten minutes. Add chicken broth and lentils: liquid should be about two inches above the lentils, and add more water or broth if not. Bring to a boil, then cover, turn the heat to low, and simmer until the lentils are soft. For me, it's usually about an hour, but I stir occasionally and watch them carefully.

While waiting for the liquid to boil, write any wishes or spells you want to include on your bay leaves. I usually just use olive oil on a fingertip, but you could also use a little balsamic vinegar as ink if you like, and toothpick makes a handy writing tool. Intent matters here more than what you use to write the word.

Add your spelled bay leaves to the pot when it's turned down to simmer. (Hey, no judgement here if your spells are misspelled or unreadable! It's not Shakespeare, it's soup: tasty, magic soup.) Chop up the rosemary, thyme, and oregano and add leaves (not stalks) to the pot. It's completely okay to use dried herbs instead, just start with a bit less because dried herbs are more potent. I've intentionally not included specific measurements here because lentil soup is truly flexible to your own tastes, which makes it easy to add extra herbs if you're in the middle of chemotherapy. Start with about a palmful of each if fresh, or a tablespoon of dried, and check the scent after they've been simmering a few minutes. Increase the amounts from there.

Dark leafy greens are a cancer superfood, and sadly I loathe the taste of kale. I find ways around it by using chard, beet greens, or even mustard greens where I can, or by finding recipes that will hide it. Lentil soup is a fabulous place to add greens because they add more bulk to make a hearty meal while providing all those delicious anti-cancer bits without drastically affecting the flavor of the soup. Chop your greens into long strips or largish chunks. I prefer two-inch strips about an inch wide, but any variation will do. The goal is to add the nutritional value and flavor of the soup, so as long as the greens are bite-sized, there's no need to be exact.

Unless you're on a low-sodium diet, lentil soup needs some salt to help draw out flavors. I start with about a teaspoon of salt and a few dashes of pepper and increase after taste tests. It's darn near impossible to fix oversalting, so if you need more, add it a pinch at a time.

When the lentils are soft and they've soaked up a good amount of the broth, the soup is done. Pull the bay leaves out and, if you can, let them dry and burn them, or put them outside in the woods. A compost pile or yard is also okay, but make sure it's not where pets could eat it by mistake. Of course, I'm practical when it comes to witchery, so if the garbage is where it needs to go, that's okay too.

Serve with crusty bread, preferably with olive oil to dip instead of butter.

LOW-ENERGY MARINARA

Tomatoes, basil, garlic, and the herbs included in Italian seasoning are all excellent nutritional and magical nutrients, and of course it would be magically beneficial for you to make your sauce from scratch with ingredients you grew yourself. But first, few of us have the space to grow our own, and second, this is a cancer treatment book. The goal here is highest beneficial results with the lowest effort and energy use, so I've included a quick "punched up" marinara recipe below which does not require hours of simmering (or even Instant Pot cooking).

Materials:
- 1 sauce pot with lid
- 1 jar organic, low sodium pasta sauce or 2 cans organic, low sodium tomato puree
- 1 can organic, low sodium tomato paste
- Olive oil (less than ½ tsp)
- 2–3 cloves garlic, smashed (or 1 tablespoon chopped or minced garlic from a jar—no judgement here!)
- ¼ cup minced onion or onion powder, to taste
- 2 tablespoons fresh basil, chopped (or 1 tablespoon dried)
- 2 tablespoons dried oregano

- 2 teaspoons dried rosemary (or about 1 tablespoon chopped fresh rosemary, sprig stem removed)
- 2 teaspoons dried marjoram
- 2 bay leaves (whole)
- Salt to taste (start with ½ teaspoons)
- ¼ teaspoons black pepper

Whether you use sauce base from a jar or make your own using tomato sauce and paste, add to the sauce pot and stir until smooth. Use the olive oil to draw a sigil for health on the bay leaf with a toothpick or your finger. You could also just write "heal" on the leaf. Add it to the pot and stir clockwise. Add garlic, herbs, and onion or onion powder (if texture is an issue for you during treatment, stick to onion powder or use a blender to smooth out your sauce before eating). Stir clockwise, focusing your intent on bringing strength and health to your body. This food supports your body in its battle against cancer and bolsters your strength to endure treatment. If you have a deity involved in your daily practice, use the stirring time to focus on a request for blessing of the food that sustains you.

Add salt and pepper, stir, and taste. Because chemo can dull your senses, you may need to add salt, but be judicious about it. If you want a little kick of spice, you could add some red pepper flakes.

This sauce can be used over noodles, zoodles, as cheesy bread dip, or over meatballs or Italian sausage. For a low-energy chicken parmigiana, bake a breaded chicken patty according to the instructions and add a slice of fresh (or a bit of shredded) mozzarella to the top of the patty for the last five minutes. Place the patty and cheese on top of noodles with marinara sauce and enjoy.

Please note while tomatoes are incredibly helpful both magically and nutritionally, particularly for cancer, they are also acidic and may not be well-tolerated.

HERBED BREAD

If you have the energy to bake bread from scratch while you're in treatment, I bow to your superpowers. I didn't, but I still wanted bakery fresh bread instead of the sort off the shelf with all the chemicals, so I compromised.

Materials:
- Frozen roll or bread dough
- Sheet pan/cookie sheet
- About 2 teaspoons olive oil

Herb options:
- Fresh or dried rosemary, thyme, and oregano (equal parts, about 1 tablespoon total), you could also add marjoram if you like it.
- 1 tablespoon fresh or dried dill
- 1 tablespoon dried "Herbs de Provence"
- 1 tablespoon fresh or dried tarragon
- ½ teaspoon flaked or sea salt
- ¼ teaspoon pepper

Thaw the dough you want to use and follow the baking instructions included to pre-heat the oven to the correct temperature. In a small bowl, combine the herbs you prefer for this loaf, salt, and pepper. Brush the top of the thawed and risen dough with a bit of olive oil, then sprinkle the herb mixture over the dough. Bake as directed.

I included the herbs and herb combinations I could taste the best during chemotherapy. Test out which ones you like best or add your own as you see fit.

INSTANT POT MASHED POTATOES

Materials:
- Instant Pot
- 1 5lb bag of your favorite potatoes (I prefer golden or red because I can leave the skin on, which is high in vitamin A)
- ¼ cup water
- Hand mixer or stand mixer
- Salt to taste (about 2 teaspoons)
- Butter to taste (optional)
- Milk (you can use soy or almond milk, just use unflavored and unsweetened…vanilla potatoes aren't tasty)

Wash the entire bag of potatoes. Remove any eyes or bruises as necessary. You can peel them or, if you like the skins, leave them on and just scrub off any dirt. Add the whole potatoes and water to the Instant Pot's fill line (if you have extra, stick them in the fridge for future use). Follow the Instant Pot's directions for cooking a full pot of potatoes. It takes about twenty minutes to pressure-cook a pot full of whole potatoes.

When the pressure-cooking cycle is complete, remove the potatoes and put them in a large mixing bowl. Mash with a handheld masher to break them into smaller chunks. Add a splash of milk (about three tablespoons) and continue mashing. When most of the large chunks are gone, add two or three pats of butter, two teaspoons of salt, and one teaspoon pepper. If possible, switch to a hand-held mixer and mix on medium until any remaining lumps are gone. If you have a stand mixer, just use the paddle attachment on a low speed to break up the whole potatoes, then add the butter, salt, and pepper and mix as noted above.

I ate a lot of mashed potatoes when my stomach was upset during chemo. It's easy to add protein by mixing in cheese and canned, rinsed black, chili, or kidney beans. Add cooked spinach, kale, Swiss chard, cabbage, or mustard greens for a version of colcannon (traditional Irish dish of mashed potatoes and cabbage). Add chili over the top or use the potatoes as a base for slow cooked beef or chicken on days you feel more adventurous.

TEA RECIPES

Honestly, I wasn't much of a tea drinker BC, but since then, I've found favorites for both physical and magical help that still use today. Adding honey to promote healing works with any of the teas I've listed below. Locally produced honey has the added benefit of helping the immune system fight allergens if you're affected by hay fever or plant allergies, because it gently familiarizes your body with local pollen. It also works wonders on a sore throat from vomiting and provides some natural sugars to help boost energy.

Bergamot (Earl Grey)
Tea for Inflammation

- A dash of ground turmeric
- A splash of milk or almond milk (optional)

Green Tea for Longevity

- A healthy dash of pomegranate juice (to taste)

Nettle Tea to Promote Healing

- Honey
- Lemon
- Turmeric

Black Tea for a Cold (Immunity Boosting)

- 2–3 teaspoons Tang (yes, the same Tang taken to space in the 1980s)
- ½ teaspoon cinnamon
- ½ teaspoon clove
- Dash of nutmeg

My oncology nutritionist advised me to drink three to four cups of tea—especially green tea—per day. Try out different additions for variety and discover which combinations work best for your palate before and after treatment. Whatever you choose, you can't really go wrong by adding tea to your diet.

Food as medicine and food as magic both follow the basic precept that we are what we eat. At some point, it's important to just get some protein and food in that will stay down while you're in treatment, so if you need to eat a single burger one day, that's okay. If you can't keep anything down but mashed potatoes for a day or two, that's also okay. Hang on, stay hydrated, and try to add as much healthy and magically beneficial food into your treatment plan as possible whenever you can.

10

Casting a Virtual Circle: Energy Raising When You Have None

There will be moments when you don't have the oomph even to sit up in bed. Extreme fatigue is a commonly known side effect of both chemo and radiation, even when you feel otherwise okay. But when you're vomiting for days at a time, not only do your muscles get sore and tender, but your energy levels plummet. The thought of doing any sort of spell work can be overwhelming.

It's possible to cast a circle from your bed or couch without moving. Mostly, it requires good visualization techniques; grounding and centering, which allows drawing some extra energy from a connection to Earth; and, of course, application of will. If you're going through treatment, you are honing your will into a strength you may not have realized you had before, because treatment is a physical and mental ordeal that forces us to stop putting energy into anything that isn't meaningful. Therefore, if you have the will to raise a bit of energy and cast a circle for yourself during treatment, you can. If you don't, you won't. I know it sounds flippant, especially when you're too exhausted to get up and get dressed, but I found it took less energy than I expected to cast a circle, and if I didn't try to hold it for too long, I was able to reabsorb most of it after I took the circle down. However, energy work requires the energy to start and focus, so it is still work that takes a toll.

First, eat something. Under normal circumstances, I usually do any sort of spirit work on a mostly empty stomach, but while you're in treatment, it's important to eat often. Yogurt, mashed potatoes, a banana, or an avocado were my go-to options during the worst of the sickness when I had trouble keeping anything down. All of them have enough sugar or starch to provide quick energy. A non-pulpy juice would also work (I stayed away from orange or grapefruit juice when nauseated, because the acidity was too harsh on my system). Set some of this aside for after you're done with your working as well, because even though you pull the energy used back into yourself, you will need a boost.

If you're doing any sort of healing or working beyond meeting with your Deity, have all of your items close by so you don't have to get up. Any workings I did while I was sick involved bay leaves or a notebook and pen. I didn't do anything with incense or candles while I was depleted, because incense usually made me nauseous and I considered candles dangerous when I couldn't guarantee I'd be able to stay awake. I spent quite a bit of time napping after casting a circle. Sleep is healing, so I figured I was healing under supervision.

Consider your position. Will you fall asleep if you're lying down? Will you get cold and therefore distracted? Are you comfortable staying still for a while without your hands or feet falling asleep? If you're sitting up, can you stay sitting with a straight back, particularly considering your overworked core muscles, or can you be bolstered and supported?

I cast a circle a few times a week, even during the worst of chemo, because it helped me feel calm. I'd lie on my bed (not between sheets, but on top) with a blanket over me so I could nap if needed. I had a yogurt cup nearby and was never without a bottle or glass of water, because dehydration is also an energy killer. I closed my eyes and started slow, deep breathing. I used the grounding and centering technique described in Chapter One to link into the earth and pull whatever energy I could. When I had no reserves, even this technique took time, which is why it's important to have eaten and to find a comfortable position.

Once I had enough energy raised, I cast my circle with the same visualization and words I used in the example earlier in this book, only instead of turning in a circle, I'd hold my bed (or bedroom) in my mind's eye and visualize the blue light sweeping in a wide line around me to whatever outer boundary I needed (sometimes the edges of the bed, sometimes more) and expanding in every direction to form a bright blue-white shield encompassing me.

CIRCLE CASTING SHORTCUTS

Materials:
- 4 stones or gems that resonate for you (one for each direction)
- 1 grounding stone: a chunk of obsidian, smoky quartz, moss agate, bloodstone, black tourmaline, or tiger's eye

Charge each of the four directional stones and the central grounding stone during ritual on a day you have a lot of energy (maybe a steroid day) or leave them under a full moon overnight.

Casting a Virtual Circle: Energy Raising When You Have None

Place the directional stones on the floor under the head, foot, and sides of your bed. Make sure they are slightly under the bed so they won't be disturbed, and they will act as permanent circle anchors you can focus on when casting a circle.

Visualize a silver line of energy connecting you to the grounding stone. The silver line extends from the stone deep into the ground, spreading roots in the earth and expanding until the line reminds you of a tree trunk, anchored and safe, feeding the grounding stone and you. See that silver cord extend from the grounding stone to you, then from you to the East stone.

See the East stone charge and fill with energy, overflowing into a line to the South stone, which fills with energy and flows to the West stone, through to the North, and back to the East. When the circle is closed, visualize it extending above and below you to create a silvery-blue globe of light around you, permeable or solid according to your own will, safely grounded through the thick trunk of the tree into the earth.

When you take the circle down, allow energy to drain down through the stones back to the obsidian grounding stone, but don't let yourself become too depleted!

Alternative Anchors:

- LED tealight candles, which can be used on your bed safely. Use as many as you like, in any colors you prefer. You could get five to ten of each of the four colors to create a specific wheel. I like yellow or pink for Air, red or orange for Fire, dark navy blue for Water, and brown for Earth.
- Four large, clean bath towels can make a small circle around you on the bed or the floor. Towels or

blankets are a lovely, cozy way to set up a comfortable "nest." Add a few drops of essential oils in appropriate scents you can still smell (and tolerate) to assist with the purpose of your working.

Of course, if you have a long cord (a cingulum in Wiccan tradition) or rope you already use for circles, that will always be an excellent option, particularly if you've used it before!

CREATING A RITUAL CORD ANCHOR

Materials:
- 3 lengths of cord, each twelve feet (about four meters) long, in three colors that are special to you. The material of the cords can vary according to your preferences, but I wouldn't use anything wider than your pinky finger
- 2 elastic hair bands

Cleanse the materials by passing through incense smoke or leave them in the sun for a day. Once the cords and bands are cleansed, crafting your cord can be done as part of a larger ritual or a standalone exercise. Whichever you choose, I recommend going outside if possible, or lighting a candle in a quiet space in the house with no distractions so you can be mindful and attentive.

Tie off one end of the cords by holding them together in a bunch in your left hand, with about two inches sticking out of the top of your fist. Make sure the three cord ends are even before binding them together with the elastic band like the bottom of a braid: place the elastic band around the ends of the cords, then pull to extend the elastic, twist once, and place over the cords again. Repeat until the elastic is too tight to add another twist.

Casting a Virtual Circle: Energy Raising When You Have None

Weave the three cords into a single braid. Take the right cord in your right hand and cross it over the center cord. This makes the right cord the center, and the center cord is now the right. Cross the left cord over the new center cord, which puts the left in the center and the center to the left. As an example, if the right cord is red, the left is gold, and the center cord is black, the pattern of crossing into the middle would be:

- Red over black so red becomes the center cord
- Gold over red so gold becomes center, red becomes left
- Black over gold, so black becomes center, gold becomes right
- Red over black so red becomes center, black becomes left

Repeat the pattern until the braid is complete. Take your time and consider what each color you've chosen means to you and why you've chosen it for this circle. Infuse the cords with your energy by visualizing warm, protective light flowing from your hands into the braid as you weave. If you would like to include requests to a god or goddess (or both) for their blessing(s), concentrate on that as you plait.

When you get to the end, you should have about nine feet of braided cord. Tie the ends off with the other elastic band. You can infuse the braid with additional energy by leaving the cord coiled under a full moon overnight, which is a low-effort way to recharge while you're in treatment.

Use the cord as an anchor of physical representation of your circle by laying it out on the floor or your bed in a closed ring, following the same clockwise (East, South, West, North) creation steps and counterclockwise (North, West, South, East) removal steps as described with the other anchors above.

I couldn't do any of my usual spell work when I was getting my first four rounds of chemo: all my energy at the time was focused on staying alive. The Red Devil is hell on the human immune system, so part of the routine is to get your infusion and have lab tests the following week to check your red and white blood cell counts. After my second round, my oncologist told me normal white cell counts should be around 11,000, and mine were at 800. Not 800,000, just 800. That was also when my energy was its lowest during the full seven months of treatment. When I say I had severe exhaustion, I mean I was afraid to take a bath because I wasn't sure I could get out of the tub. Because I couldn't keep much food down, I avoided any meat or raw vegetables and greens.

Suggestions for raising energy when you have none:
- Eat something and stay hydrated.
- Sensory-focused meditation. If you use chakras, feel free to incorporate them as you ground and center.
- Listen to emotionally uplifting, stirring music.
- Chant (even if it's a whisper, or you need breaks). If you're sitting up, it can be useful to sway with the rhythm of the chant, tap your feet, or clap.
- Walk outside and feel the wind on your face or open a window for the same (be careful to stay warm, particularly when your immune system is low).

Suggestions for spell workings when you have little to no energy:

- Ritual shower or bath with healing visualization.
- Needlepoint, cross-stitch, knitting, or some other craft you can do while sitting down. Focus on your

intention every time you work on it, while you're working on it, and don't worry if you can only do a few minutes.
- Candle magic (if you are available to keep an eye on it for safety, of course) works well if you have something magical in mind that will take more time or energy than you have in a single sitting to manifest. Burn for a few minutes per day and blow out when you're too tired to push any intent. I burned a candle daily for a month that I'd inscribed with healing symbols that resonated with me, anointed in frankincense, and rolled in healing herbs.
- Writing spells on papers or bay leaves and burning them/burying them/flushing them (assuming they're flushable), depending on the intention of the spell.
- Adult coloring books and colored pencils, markers, gel pens, or your instruments of choice. No, I don't mean pornographic "adult," I mean those intricately designed patterns you can find everywhere. Much like crafting, coloring is something you can do with intention for as long as you have the energy and set it aside when you need a nap. If you use a pattern or sigil for a spell, make sure you come back to it each time with the same intention as you fill in the pattern with your chosen colors. This is also a great way to use color magic while your energy is depleted. To set the spell, complete the pattern.

Not everyone who is a witch is a Pagan, and not every Pagan does spells. If you have or want some connection with deities, however, and you don't have the stamina to do an intricate ritual, it's okay to just do what you can. We are not required to sacrifice our wellbeing to worship. In my experience, deities are exactly the opposite, encouraging (sometimes rather insistently) self-care. I still had a connection to the Morrigan, and I took time to think at Her or talk to Her every day. Sometimes I'd do so right after I ate, and sometimes I'd meditate for a while to drop into a sacred space without expending any excess energy to cast any circle. There's a lot of background noise, like the white noise of a fan or snow on the TV, when you try to communicate with Deity outside of a sacred circle. I've always through of a circle as a silencing cone and an amplifier all at once, blocking excess crap and magnifying messages. Deep meditation can work in a similar way, requires no special tools, and if you do fall asleep, it's possible to have those conversations in dreams instead. If you can't, do little things like thinking of them fondly. Express gratitude, particularly out loud (because words are spells and naming a deity can get their attention). Ask your questions and listen for the answers. The most important thing to remember is your Deity knows what's going on. If trying is all you can do, it is enough.

11

Talismans and Stones

I have two disclaimers for this chapter, because any book on magic and Paganism needs to include stone and crystal workings. First, I rarely use stones and crystals in my practice. I have a few favorite pieces of jewelry and a few stones I've picked up over the years at shops or received as gifts, but in general I don't do much with them for myself. I tend more toward herbs, statuary, and talismans. This is the list of my favorites, but I've also included a few websites and books as resources in the bibliography for further research if stones are your thing.

Second, as with all magical tools, bits, and bobs I urge you to use what feels most right. If you're into stones and crystals, you've likely already gone through your stock and picked out the ones that are most useful to you, exactly as you should have. The following is a non-exhaustive list of useful stones and their associations, but ultimately what resonates the strongest with you will work best.

- **Agate:** courage, healing, strength, protection, love (agates are inexpensive and perfect for wearing,

including in a spell, or just having around you while you are in treatment)
- **Amber:** healing, comfort
- **Amethyst:** clear thinking and making wise decisions
- **Aquamarine:** letting go of emotional traumas/hurts, feminine energy, strength (I didn't use aquamarine at all until I was done with treatment, but it is useful to me in survivorship. Cancer is a trauma that can be difficult to release)
- **Bloodstone:** courage, healing
- **Fluorite:** visualization of cell healing, meditation assistance
- **Garnet:** protection, strength (garnet is one of my few constant gemstones because it has spoken to me since I was a child. Even before it became the center stone in my engagement and wedding rings, I wore something with garnets all the time)
- **Green Tourmaline:** soothing, boosts energy and courage (I kept a chunk on my bedside table)
- **Hematite:** grounding and centering (I keep a piece of hematite and jasper on my altar for those rare times I'm doing a formal ritual)
- **Jasper:** grounding and centering, healing, beauty
- **Jet:** protection, Earth energy, healing
- **Malachite:** strength and willpower booster (use malachite in charms and spells to help bolster your own strength and will while enduring chemotherapy and radiation treatments.)
- **Onyx:** rebuilding energy and health after a long, depleting illness (onyx jewelry is useful for me in survivorship, particularly when my energy is slow to recover)
- **Rainbow Moonstone:** healing and a sense of optimism and peace

- **Rose Quartz:** gentleness and self-love
- **Sapphire:** mental focus/will (which is so needed during treatment)
- **Snowflake Obsidian:** courage to persevere while hopeless
- **Tiger's Eye:** courage, protection

SPELL CHARM BOTTLE FOR HEALING

Materials:
- Small bottle or jar with a stopper or lid (I found lip balm-sized bottles at a local co-op, but you can order stoppered or lidded bottles online from many suppliers, including Amazon)
- An assortment of small (pencil eraser sized) stones: hematite or jasper, malachite, bloodstone, and rose quartz or rainbow moonstone
- A small piece of paper or parchment (very small, think message-in-a-bottle size: maybe ½–1 inch wide and 2 inches long)
- A pen
- A spell candle, preferably green or another color you associate with healing
- A lighter or matches

The idea here is to make a pocket-sized bottle you can take with you. Feel free to adjust this spell's materials to suit your needs: maybe you want a larger jar with different sized stones for different purposes to sit on your nightstand and help you heal while you sleep, for example.

I usually cleanse and charge my materials when I get them so they're ready to use when it's time for spell work, but if you haven't done so, please take the time to physically and metaphysically cleanse everything you're going to use, including the pen. If the material isn't washable, leave it in the sun for a few days or burn some cleansing incense, like frankincense or sage, and pass them through the incense smoke at least three times. Once cleansed, charge and attune them to you via your usual methods or, if you're too tired, keep them under your pillow or on your person for a while. I often do this with new jewelry after it's been cleansed: in my experience, wearing a new ring for a month gives it more "me" energy than a formal ritual.

When you're ready, gather your materials and prepare yourself for the work. I didn't do a full ritual because I didn't have that much energy. However, since spell work has always been more effective for me within ritual, I did cast a circle and invite my Deity to attend with a request to assist in both energy and focus. If you do the same, it may take some time as you gather your strength, so please be patient with yourself.

Cast your circle and invite your chosen attendees.

Light the candle (if candlelight is useful to you for casting your circle, you can absolutely swap the steps).

Begin with a piece of hematite or jasper because it's useful for grounding and centering. Hold the stone(s) in the palm of your left hand and cover with the palm of your right. Close your eyes and focus on your grounding exercise until you feel calm, centered, and have a bit of energy coming up from the ties you've visualized sinking deep into the earth. As that energy moves through you, call it up through your body and push it out of your right hand over the stone. In the case of hematite or jasper, the idea is to have an anchor for the spell included in the bottle, which will help hold the energy close and stabilize the working. Once you feel the stone is charged, drop it gently into the bottle.

Repeat this process for the other stones one at a time. For malachite, if you are undergoing chemotherapy or radiation to shrink your tumor(s) before surgery, energize the stone with intent to magnify the healing will and shrink tumors. For bloodstone, focus your will on the courage to persevere and keep going through your ordeal, because this is absolutely a trial that needs staying power. For rose quartz, remember to be gentle with yourself while you are trying to heal and to not push too hard or blame yourself for your illness. Foster love for your whole self, because unity of body, mind, and spirit also strengthens the healing. Drop each stone you've charged to include in your spell in the bottle.

Write your intention on your paper or parchment. This can be as simple as the word "healed" or phrase "I am healed," or as complicated as is meaningful for you. It's useful to chant whatever you choose to write as you are rolling up the paper into a small cylinder and envision the outcome as you put it in the bottle. Since the number nine is sacred to the Morrigan, I chanted *"I am healed and cancer free, as I will so shall it be"* nine times as I rolled up my little slip of paper. It doesn't have to rhyme (although I find chants are slightly easier if they have a rhythm to follow), nor does it need to be more than a single word that's meaningful to you.

Once the vial has everything you intend to include inside, secure it with the stopper or lid. To seal the spell, use the candle to drip melted wax over the stopper. Once the wax is dry, the vial can be kept near you on the bedside table, in your chemo bag with the rest of the items you bring along to infusions, in your pocket, or even around your neck if it's small enough to use as a pendant. What's important here is the charm bottle full of your intention to heal, and the certainty that you will heal, is close to you.

This chapter isn't just about the rocks we all love. I found powerful emotional and energetic assistance during treatment from talismans I carried throughout my journey. I was gifted three different bracelets from three different groups of loved ones before I started chemotherapy. Two, amusingly, had similar inscriptions. "Fuck Cancer" was inscribed on the inside of a delicate silver band, gifted to me from a group of girlfriends along with a care package, and "You Can Fucking Do This" was inscribed on the inside of a hammered silver bracelet given to me by the man I was seeing at the time I was diagnosed. The third was a lovely friendship bracelet, the tie-on middle school style made of pink and white embroidery floss, from my college girlfriends who've rooted for me in some way or another for over twenty-five years.

I wore all three every time I had a doctor's appointment, blood draw for labs, chemo treatment, or radiation appointment (I didn't wear them *in* the radiation appointment, but to and from without fail). They were all a constant reminder that not only did I have a will to live, but I also had *reasons* to live and people to fight for when I felt like it'd be easier to give up. That is powerful magic to carry along with you, and I can't recommend finding something that holds similar magic for your journey strongly enough. Cancer is full of dark places, and anything that brings you light should be included in your self-care package.

12

Accepting Help

Early on in my cancer journey, one of the biopsy nurses took me aside before I left the clinic and spoke to me with a refreshingly non-Minnesotan direct tone. "I can see you're a tough, capable woman who is fine taking care of herself, so I want you to really hear me when I say this. People who love you will want to help. Let them. You'll need it."

I'm an irritatingly independent person who assumes I'll have to take care of everything in my life on my own. Some of that is learned behavior that makes me a therapist's frustration. Some of it is likely just who I am. Giving up control of the minutiae in my life was extremely difficult, and I strongly recommend you don't follow in my footsteps.

When someone asks you what they can do for you, they aren't paying lip service. In the US, "how are you" is often dismissed as a social-contract pleasantry, not a real question, so it is often answered with some version of "good" or "fine." This is not the case when you have cancer: your friends and family members who ask how you are and what they can do for you genuinely want to help, but they don't know what you need. Cancer is scary for everyone involved; they care and are afraid you'll die and want to be there for you without intruding.

My core group of girlfriends and I had brunch to kick off the start of my journey before my first chemo session. I wore makeup, mascara on the lashes I knew would fall out with the rest of my hair, a nice dress, lipstick: all the trappings of femininity I usually avoid in favor of jeans and a t-shirt. I dressed up and made it a big event in my mind, because at that point everything felt like an event, and everything felt like it should be meaningful. So, we had a long meal, full of laughter and eggs benedict and longstanding smartass jokes, which felt normal. They did an excellent job of having a fun time without being sad, sympathetic, or pitying, and that's exactly what I needed.

They got together behind my back (those wonderful sneaks) and made a ridiculous load of frozen meals for me. It was so much food I couldn't store it in my freezer, so it had to be parceled out from my best friends' freezer over the course of the winter. I was reminded through those meals that there is healing power in the time and effort loved ones put into things for us, and when I was lonely it made me feel like I mattered, even when they couldn't visit.

That is a huge part of getting through this journey: feeling like you matter. One couple I hadn't seen in years came over on a snowy evening to clear my driveway for me because they knew I couldn't shovel. A friend dropped off toilet paper (at an appropriate distance) during the pandemic. A former coworker dropped off a bag of homemade meals and tasty snacks, including cat and dog treats for my pets, and a little surprise card with a packet of THC powder in it. The note (which I still have because it makes me laugh whenever I read it) said: "Please don't be offended, but I wanted to make sure you had some during chemo. If you'd rather not have any more, I won't bring any, but if you'd like more let me know." And that is how my retired former coworker became my surprise THC dealer during chemotherapy.

All these examples were people doing things because they had ideas on how to help, and because I was able to accept the help. I didn't say any version of "no, thank you, I'm fine," and let them do what they could.

There were a lot of folks who reached out with the bland, unspecific "if I can do anything" sentiments. Those were the ones I couldn't force myself to respond to in a meaningful way. I felt angry that they were putting the onus on me to identify what they should do, like asking me for a to-do list when I'm sick. Their sentiments felt like lip-service sympathy with no real intent to act behind it. It took me a long time to realize most of those friends, relatives, and acquaintances were genuine in their offers but didn't know what others had already done or provided. And, because I recognize the same feelings when I want to help but am at a loss for what should be done, they likely didn't want to burden me with too much company or any unwanted help.

If I had to do it over, I'd make a list of groceries I needed, housecleaning, dragging garbage bins in and out, dog walking, and just being there for company. Then I'd delegate it to someone else in my inner circle to handle coordinating help on my behalf, so I could nap. Luckily, I did have a few people in my immediate family and friends who did exactly that: my parents drove me to all my appointments, even when COVID-19 didn't allow them to sit with me for my infusions. My sister drove me to the hospital the first time I had to go to the ER. My aunt drove three hours once or twice a month to clean my house and cook for me. She'd stay a week every time and just take care of everything without asking, which was exactly what I needed.

I didn't start asking for company until it was nearly too late. I started chemotherapy the Monday before Yule in 2019.

I was still immunocompromised when COVID-19 hit in the US, so I'd been in isolation for most of the winter by the time lockdown happened. Once we were in lockdown, I couldn't safely have company at all, and I wasn't allowed to bring anyone with me to my chemo infusions. It became quite lonely. Group Zoom chats helped, but it just wasn't the same.

Help comes in many forms. If someone asks what they can do, use that excellent intuition and instinct you've spent time and energy developing in your witchcraft or Pagan practices and tell them the first thing that pops into your head (after a moment of thought to be sure it's appropriate… you wouldn't want a person who hates dogs to walk yours, after all). If nothing else, they may be able to coordinate others to help, and your constant worry about the things you aren't getting done around your house or in your life will be reduced. This reduces your stress level overall, and ultimately helps you focus on the fight at hand.

Back when I was married to my first husband, he was in a horrendous motorcycle accident. He spent a few weeks in the intensive care unit and months learning to walk again after almost dying. The social worker at the hospital told me something when we were dealing with those who loved him and wanted to help that I have used as a guideline for traumas or serious events ever since.

Vent *out*. Support *in*.

There are diagrams of this all over the internet: a series of concentric circles where the person who is dealing with the injury/illness/trauma is the center. This person only receives support and is allowed—even encouraged—to vent out to any of the other circles. The second ring is the patient's spouse, closest friend, or confidant: the primary caregiver. They may be a parent or sibling, but it is not meant to represent the immediate family, just the person/people most responsible for daily and intimate physical or emotional care. The person in this ring accepts venting from the patient, sends support to the patient, and does *not* vent to the patient. This person vents out to the next circle of support, and accepts their support back in.

The closer you are to the person handling the injury or illness, the more support you receive and less venting you handle. This prevents the people enduring treatment—and their immediate caregivers—from having to comfort those who should be supporting them with their extra energy. If you like spoon theory better, your spoons (or bandwidth) for supporting others decreases the closer you are to the center, because your focus is on the person/people in the central ring(s).

There are some tricky emotional pitfalls associated with the circles of support theory, though, particularly for empathetic or intuitive people (like witches) that are worth mentioning. If part of how you've built meaning into your life is based on helping others, on being an advice-giver, priest or priestess, or just that empathetic ear to your friends and loved ones, suddenly getting cut off from those energies can feel like abandonment. If your emotional and mental wellbeing needs include some level of supporting your loved ones, do so. Witches and Pagans are often very self-aware of their limitations; pay attention to your own and don't overextend, even when you think you need to. Your primary focus needs to be survival, which means a certain amount of hoarding energy, even if that's far from normal for you.

Children present a whole different set of requirements, and I would never tell you to ignore your kids' need for reassurance and comfort. Their importance just makes the rest of the rings so vital because the patient and caregiver will need as much help as people can offer.

Oncology offices are experts at finding volunteer assistance for patients and patients' families, whether that's some form of therapy, practical help with chores, financial resources, or childcare. It's worth asking them about local resources. Gilda's Club, started by the late Gilda Radner, has chapters in major cities all over the United States. They specialize in cancer support of all sorts for the entire family: there are programs for cancer patients as well as their families and caregivers, including programs specifically for children trying to handle a parent's cancer. If you're in the States and looking for a place to start outside of your oncology office's advice, I'd start there.

Accepting help can be tricky when you aren't used to it, and cancer brings people out of the woodwork who want to help. If you aren't used to having help for whatever reason, it may be difficult to remember that it's not only expected but preferred that you say yes: let people help you. A brain that usually responds "no, I'm fine thank you" to offers of assistance will need some retraining.

I found it easiest to charm one of my favorite pieces of jewelry as a visual reminder that I could say yes when someone offered help.

CREATE A "YES" TALISMAN

Materials:
- A favorite bracelet, ring, or necklace
- Candle and matches or lighter (can be any color candle: maybe yellow for inspiration, or orange for resilience, or even blue for positive mental health)

Optional:
- Cleansing incense (whatever variety you prefer)

Begin by settling yourself in a quiet space, then ground and center. If you choose to cast a circle and call your deities, do so now.

Accepting Help

If the jewelry you wish to charm is something you wear often, you may not want to pass it through cleansing incense because it's already attuned to you. However, doing so dedicates the piece as a talisman reminding you that you are worthy of help and should accept help when offered, if it's useful. To cleanse, light incense such as frankincense or your favorite scent, then pass the bracelet, pendant, or ring through the smoke three times.

Light the candle, close your eyes, and take three deep breaths. Think about why it is difficult for you to accept help: are you especially stubborn or stoic (like me)? Do you fiercely protect your independence? Does help make you feel weak or incapable?

Hold the jewelry in your palm. Think about saying "yes" to an offer and the reasons why you want to be more accepting of help. Create a path in your mind to analyze and identify whether you should say yes by visualizing the following questions:

1. Is it a useful and specific offer (clean your kitchen, take the garbage bins out for you, shovel snow)?
2. Is the offer asking *you* to do anything (make a list, give someone something to do)? If you have a list pre-made, can you hand them the list and say "sure, I could use anything on this list if you want to help out"? If you don't, this may be a moment to answer with a "thank you, let me consider that" or "I'll keep you in mind, thanks."
3. What does your gut say? If you want the help and have feelings (guilt, not wanting to be a nuisance, fear someone will think less of you) or habits (control issues, lack of delegation) that would normally prevent you from saying yes, trust your gut. Take the help.

4. Assume the person who wants to help is trying to be kind, even if their offer isn't what you need or mistakenly puts the effort in your hands to figure out something for them to do. You aren't obligated to take their help, and you aren't obligated to respond to them in any particular way, but it is useful to remember that even unhelpful offers usually come from good intentions.

When you finish this meditation, look at the jewelry in your palm and focus your will and intention on it. Infuse the metal, stones, or patterns on the piece with a reminder that people want to help you, you are worthy of receiving help, and you don't have to do this alone.

Complete your ritual, opening the circle and dismissing any attendees with gratitude. Blow out your candle and put on the charmed jewelry. After this ritual, wear the bracelet, ring, or necklace as often as possible throughout treatment: it is a visual reminder that you have made an intention to be more receptive to assistance when it shows up in your life, at least during this difficult time.

Sometimes during cancer treatment, the sheer stupidity that dribbles out of people's mouths can be astounding. Our society has done such a good job of sanitizing death and suffering, sweeping it into hospices or hospitals, that most people don't handle critical illness or the potential of death well. Curiosity and fear make them inappropriate. I can't count the number of people who asked quite invasive questions they'd never dream of asking before cancer. I mean, the list of folks who can reasonably ask about how much weight I'd lost, or whether I threw up all the time, or could I still have sex (yes, someone asked that) is incredibly short.

Of course, those people would never ask because they know me well enough not to.

At the other end of that spectrum are the people who tell you all about the horrors their first cousin twice removed faced when they were going through treatment for stomach cancer, or how their grandpa got Stage IV lung cancer even though he never smoked. Those stories usually ended with the patient dying or "but they got better and so will you." Unhelpful.

I think fear is the driving force behind the awkward attempts to connect because it's uncomfortable to look in the eyes of a person you know who's in a life-threatening crisis. It's too close to mortality, like death might accidentally rub off if they get too close. But most people, even the awkward ones, are trying to be empathetic. They want to be supportive, but they're also, perhaps understandably, relieved it isn't happening to them, or they're reminded of someone else who had to go through it. If you can muster it, I recommend looking at these occurrences with as much humor as possible, and remember their reaction isn't personal. Or you can do what I did and keep a log or list of all the stupid shit people say while you're at your worst. If nothing else, it makes a good reminder that overall, humans are amusingly inept in many ways (a statement I include myself in, which makes me feel more like a person than a science experiment).

What about the Christian folk—friends or family or strangers—who offer to pray for you? Pagan perspectives and traumas on deity can be so extensive and different that there is no right or wrong answer. Your reaction to the offer may fall anywhere on a wildly varied range of emotions, not always predictable. If your first instinct is positive, tell them thank you and let 'er rip. If it's negative, it's okay to say you're not a Christian and it makes you uncomfortable, but you can't control whether they do it anyway. In general, I took offers to pray for me by Christians the same way I would any other Pagan who doesn't share my calling for my Goddess: positive thoughts expressed to Deity are positive thoughts, no matter whose face Deity wears.

I did have an occasion or two to say my version of "no thanks." If it seemed genuinely caring, I was all about someone sending a little extra spiritual boost into the universe on my behalf. If it seemed like the offer was a condescending "I'll pray for you because cancer is a punishment for turning away from God," I told that person to fuck right off into the sun.

I lost my romantic partner during chemo. (Ugh, that's still a shitty thing to write, even years later. Some scars last a long time.) He'd made it through diagnosis and surgery, for the most part, but after Yule I didn't see him again until Valentine's Day, which was a short and uncomfortable visit. When I was afraid to start chemo and lose my hair, he used to joke that he'd shine my bald head until he could use it as a crystal ball. Unfortunately, reality proved he couldn't even look at me much after he saw me that sick on Yule. He stayed in contact via text, but when I went to the emergency room (twice) during treatment, he avoided both the hospital and any visits at home. By the time lockdown for COVID-19 came around, it was clear he couldn't deal with me or my disease. It took a while, but eventually he admitted he thought I'd die. So, his response to supporting a woman he claimed to love while she was dying (I was not dying, for the record) was to bail.

Oncology doctors and nurses told me the harsh, unfair truth: this is horrendously common for women, and almost never happens to men, going through chemotherapy. According to a US study conducted in the early 2000s the divorce or separation rate among cancer patients is 11.6%, but it jumps to a 20.8% rate if the patient is a woman. Divorce or separation is only a 2% rate if the patient is a man. The percentages only reflect straight couples and don't include other romantic relationship compositions (especially poly, gay and lesbian, trans, intersex, and other LGBTQIA people and relationships), so please take the results with the salty cisgendered heterosexual bias presented in the study.

Of course, these statistics depend on culture and timing and the subject group, and there are likely more studies in progress that may have changed the stats since I wrote this book. But the sheer number of support sites for breast cancer patients whose partners bailed during treatment is a hefty stack of evidence. In case you need it, SurvivingBreastCancer.org has articles specifically about relationship support, including links to other websites that may be useful. The site address is included in the bibliography.

When I asked for some common examples, the nurses at the oncology clinic commented on how often men would ask inappropriate things like "but when can she cook (or clean, do laundry, work, have sex, take care of the kids) again, I can't keep eating cereal?" They always asked in front of the woman going through treatment, as if her fight for her life was upsetting not because she may die, but because suddenly he must do some of the household management. It's disturbingly easy to find anecdotes like this on social media, too. At my most absolutely and objectively generous, I can see a way these offensive questions come from feeling useless in the face of a sickness they can't fix. But the unspoken end to those kinds of questions is always "so I don't have to," which disgusts me on every level. Rage and despair due to a romantic partner fleeing when you need them the most is not a side effect of cancer treatment the medical team talks about, but they nod with the sad and resigned expression of someone who's seen it too many times when you tell them about it.

If it happened to you, I am so very sorry, and please know their leaving was *not* your fault at all. It's their failing as a partner, not yours. If your partner is a wonderful and supportive caretaker while you are fighting for your life, you have my enthusiastic support to feel relieved, happy, and even smug while reading this. I love that you are supported.

Cancer is shitty to deal with for you and your loved ones. As with any major trauma in a person's life, cancer is the sieve through which your true family and friends separate themselves from those who don't matter. When the ones who can't hack it leave, let them. They've proven who they are to you and to themselves. Could you curse them? Sure. Is it worth your energy when they know they've failed? Debatable.

Also, do you want another spiritual link to that person? I believe cursing creates a negative tie to a person who has proven they aren't good for you and don't have your best interests in mind, so I avoid cursing in general and stick to severing all ties. If healing your heart's hurts from things that happened during treatment requires you to do some sort of ritual redress, I wish you all the luck in letting that hurt go so you can move on, but I have no curses to share. To me, they aren't worth my closely guarded energy reserves.

However, a ritual fire to help let go of intentional and unintentional wrongs done during cancer is always useful.

FIRE RITUAL FOR RELEASING WRONGS

Materials:
- Fire (outside or fireplace) or cauldron, fireproof bowl, or pot
- Candle (if not fire)
- Glass of water (blessed is great, but not required)
- Pen or marker
- Dried bay leaves
- Paper
- A flat surface

Ideally this ritual would be done with an outside fire, whether a bonfire or firepit. But that may not be possible, and indoor fireplaces are harder to find (particularly in Minnesota), so this ritual is just as effective with a candle and cauldron if you don't have access to a fire or don't have the oomph to start one.

Light your fire (or candle) and watch the flames as you ground and center yourself with long, deep breaths. When you are calm and feel within your own sacred space, think of the specific things said or done that caused your heart and mind harm. Look at them from a distance and identify the feelings they bring up inside you. Remember you do not have to feel this way. Remember that people hurt people they love through indifference, ignorance, fear, and selfishness, and those are not hurts you are required to carry. This is not about forgiveness of their behavior, but deciding to let go of the hurts so you do not continue the injury when you remember their acts.

Ball up all those feelings and push them through your hand into the pen. Write each act or comment that hurt you on bay leaves and allow the feelings to flow through the pen to the leaf. Bay leaves help with healing, protection from harmful energies, and wishes. I put a single thing on each leaf so I can focus on one at a time, but you can also write it on a slip of paper if you need more room, then fold a leaf in the paper.

Take the bay leaf in your hand and read the writing out loud, followed by:

> *"This caused me hurt and harm, and I burn it now to release myself from the ties it created. So begins healing."*

Put the leaf into the fire or hold it to the candle until it's ablaze and drop it in the cauldron or fireproof bowl to burn to ash.

Repeat this process until your list is complete and burned away. Take a deep breath and raise your arms above your head. As you exhale, feel the lightness after the weights of others' actions are reduced to ash. If you burned your wishes for healing in a bowl inside, add the ashes to your glass of water, take it outside, and bury the mixture so it can be cleansed by the earth. Or flush the water and ash down the toilet.

In survivorship I still must parse out my energy carefully, so I use this ritual often. It keeps my mind and heart as clear as possible from the casual and directed harm caused by others. It's practical, easy, and allows me to act without impeding anyone else's agency.

You know that phenomenon when you buy a new blue car and suddenly you see your exact car in your exact color everywhere, even though you could swear you'd never seen them before and had no idea they were so popular? Suddenly, inspirational cancer stories showed up in every magazine about chemo patients who wrote a book or planned out their new restaurant from the ground up or learned a new language because they were "just lying around anyway."

Stories about supermoms who balanced work, chemo, and their families without dropping any of those work/dishes/homework/kid sports/costumes/holiday/spouse-date balls were in every social media feed. And don't they all look so fresh and beautiful in their fully made-up faces and adorable hats to cover their bald heads? How exactly do they still have eyebrows and lower eyelashes (there aren't false eyelashes for the lower lids, FYI, so no matter what it looks slightly weird) and clear skin? Aren't they so brave and strong and inspirational? Of course, they *were* brave and strong and inspiring and beautiful.

It was *infuriating* and depressing.

I had no energy during chemotherapy. None. The mild cold I had before starting chemo morphed into an evil combination of bronchitis and double sinus infection that sapped every ounce of oomph and chapped my nose to boot. I was too sick to leave my house for the two full months of the Red Devil other than chemo appointments. I wore a mask, terrified of getting another virus, long before COVID-19 hit.

I lost forty pounds in those first eight weeks, which oncology will tell you is not ideal. Cancer medical teams don't want you to lose weight during treatment, even when you're significantly overweight, because your immune system needs you to eat. I spent most days that winter under blankets on my couch or in bed, doing little more than going ten steps to the bathroom to vomit or twenty steps to the kitchen to find something soft enough to eat that wouldn't scrape my esophagus when it came back up. Ninety percent of my waking life revolved around whether I could find something with protein or vitamins that I could keep down between the reminders to take the next round of medication.

On top of that, all the messaging from the media was that breast cancer treatment is both awful and somehow no big deal. As though I, as a woman, should just be able to fold this into my daily duties and accomplish even *more* during this time because, well, I'm just lying around anyway. The expectation is clear that if you aren't making use of your time off while you're in the chemo chair, you're failing. If you aren't creating or producing while you're at home on medical leave, you're failing. If you aren't managing all your familial commitments and making everyone around you feel better about *your* cancer and mitigating their fears, you're failing. Basically, if you aren't superwoman, you suck at cancer, and you are not allowed to just rest.

The entire point of this chapter is to tell you this is *complete horseshit*.

I don't care if you have Stage 0 (staging is based on tumor grade, lymph node status, whether the cancer has spread to other parts of the body, and various hormonal factors. The Susan G. Komen website has excellent information about how pathology determines stage, and Stage 0 is still breast cancer), Stage IV, or anything in between. *You are allowed to rest.* Cancer is an all-encompassing terror-bomb in your life, and it's okay if you can't handle it all with perfect aplomb. It's okay if you need help with your kids. It's okay to lean on your partner. It's okay to lean on your friends and family. And, most importantly, you are not obligated to produce or create anything while your body is trying desperately to stay alive.

If you need something to keep your mind busy while your body rests so you plan a garden, a new business, or a book, I say more power to you. That is incredible, and I'm in awe of your ability to focus. But if you can't—if you're like me and just can't muster enough bother for anything but basic survival for those two months—that's okay too.

Everything in American culture pits women against each other, and it starts in early childhood. Mommy wars, body shaming, slut shaming, queen bees…it's all garbage rooted in a sense of insecurity and competition we're taught all our lives. Cancer is not a competition, and you are not required to do, be, or accomplish anything in your cancer journey beyond what you choose to accomplish. I won't say that your only accomplishment is to live, because that assumes survival is possible for everyone, and the truth is that sometimes we just make the best choices we can with the energy we have left to dole out. So, if you get inspired by all the "this is what I created when I was doing chemo" stories, awesome. If you don't, that's okay. You have all the permission to just be.

If you're lucky enough to have some sort of medical leave available to you, take it. I know not everyone does, and in this country it's a huge luxury to have medical insurance all, much less disability leave through your job. So, if you have that available to you, take it, because every bit of help you have access to is worth it. I tried to work through the first few weeks of treatment and it was a huge mistake. I'm a business analyst at an insurance firm, so most of my job involves some sort of problem solving or documentation, and "chemo brain," the slow-thinking fog that comes along with chemotherapy and associated medication, is real. I took the first three months of 2020 off, and I really think if I hadn't, I may not have kept that position because I could not perform my usual duties at all.

By the third month into 2020, I was on Taxol instead of the Red Devil and felt well enough to go back to work in April. Looking back, I do not recommend going back early. I was worried I'd lose my job if I didn't come back as soon as possible because I'd only been there ten months before I was diagnosed, but those first few months back while I finished chemotherapy and radiation were a waste. It took twice as long for me to do normal work, and often I'd lie down for a twenty-minute nap at lunch and wake up three hours later. My boss and team were all incredibly kind, and I will always be grateful to them for their support, but ultimately it would've been better for me *and* for my team if I'd stayed out and let someone take over until treatment was finished. It takes longer than you think to recover. Take what time you can. As of writing this, I've been done with treatment for three and a half years, and I still have bouts of brain fog and exhaustion. Cancer isn't easy on your body, mind, or spirit: it's good to give yourself grace and be patient about healing.

SPELL TO GIVE YOURSELF GRACE

Grace is one of the most difficult things to give ourselves. It's so much easier to blame ourselves, to abuse ourselves with our inner thoughts and feelings of insecurity or inadequacy, than it is to allow space for our own humanity and needs. Humans aren't superheroes. Humans fail. Humans need rest, and love, and patience. Most of us seem perfectly capable of allowing for mistakes, growth, and rest for those we love, but we don't express that same love to ourselves because so much of this society is based on a layer of guilt if you need to pause (or stop) contributing.

While I'm neither a neuroscientist nor licensed counselor, my own therapist once told me that our brains don't hear negative modifiers. Saying "I will not do" something doesn't help your brain rework long established habits, because it drops the "not" from the statement. For some reason, many people find it difficult to say positive things to themselves about themselves. This would be an important aspect of self-love to develop under normal circumstances, but during cancer treatment it becomes vital because the constant cycles of exhaustion, sickness, and worry wears down even the most positive person, and despair can lead to giving up.

If you've picked up this book because you've already established yourself as a Pagan of some flavor, you have likely already done some of this work to see yourself in the best light possible. That means you may have a developed mantra or spell for grace, even if that's not what it's specifically called. If you already have a ritual or spell that works for you, it's a useful healing tool to perform daily.

If you don't have your own, my good friend Tony, the best chant- and spell-writer in my circle, has offered the following chant. It can easily be used as a fully ritualized spell if you have the energy, but it can also be quietly whispered while you're in the bath or shower, or while lying in bed, or shouted at the sky. It's an excellent sentiment to repeat while on a walk outside or another form of moving mediation.

If you can, light a candle and watch the flame for a while as you breathe deeply. Cast your circle and acknowledge your Deity in the sacred space outside of time. When you feel settled and ready, recite the following lines at least three times:

> "*I breathe in the love from those closest to me and gain the warmth I need to heal.*
> *I breathe out the anger that does not serve me in the journey that I am on.*
> *I breathe in the acceptance of my circle and gain strength for the fight before me.*
> *I breathe out the intolerance I hold for my flaws and shortcomings, for they too are a part of me and deserving of love.*
> *I breathe in the grace afforded me by the universe and increase the knowledge that I have value in the grander scheme of existence.*
> *I breathe out the presumption that I am unworthy of healing.*

*I am worthy of the blessings I have been bestowed in
the past, those which arrive now,
and those in my future.
In this way I increase my healing threefold and find my
way through challenges to the other side of this path."*

(Chant by Tony Cruikshank)

Yes, the words should be said out loud. I know not all of us (including me) like saying things out loud about ourselves, even in sacred space while alone but for our gods, but words are powerful spells and ideally should be voiced aloud to the universe to set them.

Give yourself the gift of grace and patience while you heal. For what it's worth, I think you're doing a fantastic job, and you don't have to do anything more. Whatever you're doing to get through cancer treatment is enough.

13

Grieving and Facing Death

"We must be willing to let go of the life we planned so as to have the life that is waiting for us."

—Joseph Campbell

I refer to my life now with a BC/AC delineation, because the day I found out I had cancer, the woman I was before diagnosis died. My meat suit betrayed me, and all the plans I'd made for the future burned to ash in a sickly cancerous flame when the clinic called. In that moment, it didn't matter whether I was curable or not: everything stopped in my world.

A cancer diagnosis (or any life-changing critical illness) is a trauma that forever changes you. The person you planned to be before your diagnosis dies with the words "you have cancer." In the flurry of doctor's appointments, surgical consults, MRIs, biopsies, and planning that all eat time and fill space in your head for those first few weeks, it often feels like there's no room to consider that the life you had in mind for yourself is gone.

It's gone, and grieving that loss follows the same pattern as all grief, hitting at unexpected and often inconvenient moments. I am so, so sorry.

A heaviness of heart and soul lurks beneath the distractions of activity, waiting until you're alone in the dark when everyone else is asleep. It's hiding in those quiet 3 a.m. moments when you can't keep the tornado of fear and grief locked in the basement of your mind anymore. And that grief is an important thing no one talks about during treatment. You have lost your old life: even if you carry on every day with normal things and pretend everything is the same, it isn't. You have cancer, and you'll always worry about cancer even after it's gone; an innocence of mortality is lost when a person is diagnosed with a life-threatening illness, the same way it is anytime a person brushes against Death. All of those "I'll get to that someday" events in your life get sifted through a simple yes/no lens: "*yes*, I'm going to do that" or "nope, doesn't matter at all." Sadly, some of those "somedays" are taken from you, even after slotting them high up in that yes column.

The lost possibility that hurt me the most was surprising and unexpected. I was forty-two years old, divorced, in a long-term but not cohabitating relationship with someone who'd had a vasectomy years before we dated, and I'd avoided having children all my life. My ex-husband never wanted children of his own, and for years, that was okay with me. In my thirties, I started to think it might be nice to have a baby, but I wasn't driven enough to go have one alone (before or after my divorce). I had opportunities, but I still held out some deep desire to have a real partner for parenting. So, I chose not to use a fertility clinic, adoption agency, or even a one-night stand. By the time I hit my early forties, I thought I'd accepted a childless life: I was happy in my relationship, happy with my job, and generally happy with my free lifestyle.

Because my breast cancer was hormone positive, my own body's estrogen and progesterone fed the tumors. That means from the time I finished radiation to whenever I hit menopause, I will be on a hormone blocking medication, Tamoxifen, to prevent a recurrence. Both my oncologist and gynecologist strongly recommend I never get pregnant, meaning they said, "absolutely *not*." I'm technically still able to have children, but I'm not supposed to; the risk of recurrence is too high.

But I'd already decided not to be a mom, so why the hell was it devastating to have that option removed? Suddenly, I had no choice: I felt like all the potential I had to change my mind was stolen from me. I grieved a secret dream of having a family of my own so deeply I couldn't express it until after active treatment was over. I still grieve it.

This is where I would share a spell with you that fixes your grief for the losses you are forced to bear with cancer. I wish to all the gods that I had that spell for us both. Grief is its own beast, and it sneaks up on you when you're unprepared, or when you thought you were done with it. There is time, though, to grieve the old life.

Moving forward in a new life, however that looks and however long that is, doesn't mean forgetting who you were BC. Cherish the person you used to be, because they got you where you are now. There is still joy and purpose to be found, no matter how long your after-cancer life is expected to be. I am still grieving the life I thought I'd have, but it doesn't stop me from transitioning to the new one. I am angry, sad, and scared often. I am still here. I am still going.

No treatment plan is without risk, and while chemotherapy is commonly included in a cancer treatment plan, it isn't guaranteed to succeed, nor is it gentle. Sometimes it seems like the time from diagnosis to the time you ring the bell is one long exercise in facing mortality. Included in the packets of information I got from my oncology team was a health directive form, because death lurks everywhere during treatment.

I went to the ER twice during chemo: once for a bleeding throat, and once after the first week of Taxol because my body just gave out. I was celebrating the first week of what was a more tolerable chemotherapy by having homemade chicken noodle soup at my best friends' house. Ben and Sarah had been switching off between supporting me and taking care of their new little one. Months prior, he'd hung out with my mom in the hospital waiting room and stayed at my house as the responsible adult for that first twenty-four hours after the anesthesia when I'd had my lumpectomy. This time, he was out of town ice fishing, and it was Sarah's turn to watch over me, although that wasn't the intent of our girls-only evening.

It was supposed to be for soup and a relaxing visit for the three of us: Sarah, me, and their one-year-old. I remember Sarah handing me the baby and we were chatting about something, then I felt a little nauseated and woozy, my body going alternately hot and cold. I said something like "take the baby." And then I was dreaming, but I can't remember the dream.

From her perspective, I was fine one minute, then I handed her the baby and sat rigidly in my chair, eyes open, not breathing for about ninety seconds. Naturally, that scared the shit out of her. When I came to, I didn't remember the weird passing out and just felt a little sick, so I got up to go lie on the couch and woke up on the floor in the kitchen, because, apparently, when I stood up, I promptly passed out like a ton of bricks. I only avoided a collision between the counter and my noggin because Sarah was able to catch and guide me down.

She called an ambulance because every time I sat up, I'd pass out again, although I was mostly fine lying down. I made it all the way to forty-two-and-a-half years old before I had to be carried out on a stretcher by two lovely paramedics and a cop (also, I am six feet tall and not a light woman, so I'm still thoroughly amazed they carried me out of there). It turned out to be some sort of reaction to the Taxol, and much like the other weird side effects I had, my oncologist essentially logged it, shrugged, and said since I know the warning signs, I should be okay doing normal life things like driving, just as long as I pull over if I feel that hot/cold/nausea combination again.

Not super comforting, is it? Chemo specifically, and cancer treatment in general, changes the way you live your daily life. It seems like there's constantly some new change, challenge, pain, side effect, or fear to be faced, treated, and cataloged. The awful truth is there is no guarantee that the next weird scary thing treatment does to your body will be fixable, and the next ambulance ride could be the last. Cancer treatment is a complicated dance with death, even in the best circumstances.

Norm McDonald (before he passed from cancer himself) famously said he hates it when someone's obituary says they "lost their battle" with cancer, because it's a lie: if you die of cancer, you've killed your cancer, too.

What about those of us who know cancer will be the death of us because there is no cure available, just ways to medically put off the inevitable? Are those patients still battling, or are they slowly coming to a delicate state of balance for as long as they can, living with this new state of being and managing their best, much like someone diagnosed with other incurable lifelong illnesses?

About a year after I finished treatment, I was contacted by an acquaintance for advice, because she'd just been diagnosed with a different form of breast cancer. Two years later, despite all her traditional and experimental treatments, she passed away. When they learned her prognosis was incurable, she and her loving husband took their kids on a family vacation before ending her treatment and planning for her end-of-life care. She was three years younger than me. During her funeral, I thought for a long time about why I lived, the unfairness of it all, how her fight for survival evolved into acceptance, and her drive to make her transition as easy on her husband and children (and herself) as she could. There is no wrong approach, only the approach that works best for you and your loved ones.

This can be hard, terrifying, depressing stuff to talk about, even if you have established concepts of death and the afterlife. The plain truth is that not all of us will be cured. Not all of us will ever be finished with chemo. Death comes everyone eventually, and complications can happen even during routine treatments. Thinking about the "what-if" scenarios is encouraged by oncology: my doctor and nurse practitioner strongly encouraged me to consider creating my living will and medical directives, so everyone knew what I wanted if it became necessary. Even in death, there are choices to be made if you want to hang on to your agency.

Late stage and incurable cancers also prompt pharmaceutical companies and researchers to come knocking. When all other treatments have failed, they hope you're willing to be in a trial for some new medications or treatments for your type of cancer. Often, this doesn't mean a miraculous last-ditch cure for you, but rather an invitation to help someone else beat the same thing in the future. It is another choice to make with no right or wrong answer.

The choices presented when facing and accepting our own mortality, particularly when it feels imminent, are part of a unique ordeal most of us just aren't prepared for. Sometimes the best we can do is follow Gandalf's advice from *The Lord of the Rings*: "All we have decide is what to do with the time that is given to us." (Tolkien, 1988, p. 60)

SIMPLE CANDLE MAGIC SPELL FOR ACCEPTANCE

Materials:
- Matches or a lighter
- A tealight or small taper beeswax candle
- A journal or notebook
- A pen or pencil

Acceptance is a process, not an instant, castable result. That's why it's the last stage of many forms of change, including processing death. Unfortunately, the only way out is through, so at least a couple of times a week, take an hour to light your candle and journal or free write. You can do this inside sacred space if you have the energy to cast a circle, or you can take the example questions below one at a time as you are ready.

Inscribe the candle with sigils if you are inclined to do so, anoint it with a purifying oil like frankincense, or use one infused with herbs (make sure the scent doesn't make you nauseated). Focus your attention on the flame as it burns and ground and center yourself before you start to write. Be mindful of what feelings bubble up and feel them flowing out of you through the ink or graphite onto the paper. As with any long-term candle magic, blow the candle out when your exercise is completed for that session. There is no time limit for this exercise: when your candle has burned to the base, you can always get another candle and keep going. Some questions and prompts you might consider include:

1. What is my biggest fear about my own death?
2. Who will I miss most? If I knew I was going to die tomorrow, what would I want them to know?
3. *Who will miss me the most?* Consider how much you are loved by those to whom you matter.

4. What about my death would be a relief?
5. What haven't I finished which matters to me?
6. How do I feel about preparing things legally, like a medical directive or living will? Are there financial concerns after death that I worry about? Write about that worry, because working through the feeling will help to focus next steps to removing those concerns.
7. If I won't be here for my children, what do I want them to know about me? What lessons do I want to pass along?
8. Make a list of "just in case" letters to children and family members, and work on those letters when there is energy for it. Note: if you decide you need this particular exercise, make sure the letters are hidden from loved ones until you're ready for them to read them, or designate someone to dole them out appropriately. If you're going through treatment with every expectation of survival, you may want to write them as an exercise in acceptance and just set them aside.
9. I am so fucking angry. This is completely unfair. I have things to do and people to love.
10. I feel so alone.

When you're done with the session for that day, close your circle (if you've cast one), thank the deities in attendance (if you've invited them), and gently blow out your candle. Push your shoulders forward, then raise them up near your ears, pull them back, and let them drop. Repeat twice. Let the tension you've been holding sink into the earth through your grounding. Close your eyes and take three deep breaths: inhale to the count of five, hold for a count of five, and exhale to a count of five. After the third breath, open your eyes. Drink some water and, if you can, go eat something.

The feelings around our mortality are a complex, swirling mess to unravel, and some feelings may cause secondary reactions like shame or fear. Nobody can see this except you: write about those feelings as they come up, too. Over time, you will ideally start to feel at peace with mortality and discover what unfinished business presses upon you while you're in treatment.

PART III

SURVIVORSHIP AND REBIRTH

14

CELEBRATING

If you've come to this chapter because you want to know what's next, you've either made it through chemo, radiation, surgery, and whatever other trials were placed in your path to killing the cancer within you, or you expect to do so. First, congratulations are in order, because looking at survivorship is truly a new beginning and I'm so happy for you!

There were two days that I felt truly well and done with cancer: the first happened when I walked out of my final chemotherapy infusion. Out of consideration for the patients whose chemo has no end date, my clinic didn't have a bell to ring. Instead, I said my goodbyes and went out to my car, alone because it was May 2020, mid-COVID-19 lockdown, so I wasn't allowed to have anyone with me. I cried in the driver's seat for a while in sheer relief and some self-pity for hitting this milestone alone. Then I got myself some fancy coffee, which I could finally taste again, and went home.

Later that day, a few of my closest friends drove an obnoxiously awesome caravan of honking cars and hollering family outside my house (again, because we were all in COVID-19 lockdown) and delivered a porcelain bell, which

I promptly smashed on my driveway in triumph. It felt glorious. I still have the dove from the end of that bell in the same box as my "fuck cancer" bracelet talismans. Finishing chemotherapy is a monumental accomplishment, and you deserve to celebrate it in whatever manner fits you best. Culturally, many of us (particularly women) are conditioned not to celebrate ourselves. Do it anyway.

The second time I felt celebratory was after my twenty-fourth and final round of radiation. This one didn't have a big noisy parade that disrupted the neighborhood, partially because I was still exhausted. I felt jubilant when I walked out of the hospital the last time. It was June 2020, so I took the day off work and napped in my hammock in the sun for the afternoon, determined to enjoy every drop of relief that the prior eight months were finally over.

It's important to celebrate your wins, to open yourself up to amazing new opportunities that present themselves, and to live in the moment as much as you can. Breast cancer is a terrible ordeal for you and your caregivers, and there is truly no way out but through. But you have the support of your loved ones, your medical team, and the Universe backing you up.

Time slows down when your milestones are getting through a day without vomiting, finishing the final round of the worst of chemo, or taking the bandages off after surgery. Celebrate those wins however you can and include your loved ones whenever you can. Cancer is full of horrendous moments, so anything you can do to relieve some of the stress and pressure will help your spirit stay resolved and your attitude resilient. Gratitude for small wins also helps with this. Light a candle and say thank you to your chosen Deity when you've had a good day or won a fight to keep yogurt down. Tell yourself "I did it!" when you take that short walk to the mailbox.

RITUAL OF GRATITUDE

Materials:
- Milk, for abundance and offering
- Honey, for healing and offering
- Spoon
- A glass or bowl
- White candle (pillar, tealight, or taper in a candle holder)
- God/dess and quarter candles
- Matches or a lighter
- Incense or smudge bundle you prefer for purification and renewal (I use frankincense, juniper, or dragon's blood)
- Journal or paper
- Writing utensil

Find a space where you are alone and at peace. This ritual can be done inside or out. Ground and center, cast a circle, and call quarters as you see fit. Light your quarter candles as you call.

Invite your Deity or Deities to the space, and light the God/dess candle as appropriate.

Light the white candle and say:

"I passed the trial, I crossed the ford. My path stretches before me, renewed as I am renewed."

Reflect in the sacred space about your cancer journey, the trials you faced, and the support you received from friends, relatives, medical teams, and deities. Take the time to consider the gravity of what you've just been through and any help you had to get here.

Write down your thoughts and feelings about what you endured during cancer treatment, and what is to come in survivorship. Take note of any fears or worries you carry now that you're moving into this new phase of post-treatment life.

Light your incense or smudge stick and bathe yourself and your space in the smoke. You are no longer the person you were before cancer, and your future lies before you. Take deep breaths and focus your energy on embracing the new life you pass into as a survivor.

Consider any help you've had from your specific deities as you pour the milk and a good dollop of honey into a glass or bowl. Mix the offering of abundance, purity, and gratitude clockwise with your spoon and take time to thank your deities. Feel free to add anything specific to your deities to the milk and honey mixture so it becomes more personal to Them. For example, I added a shot of good Irish whiskey into mine for the Morrigan.

Hold the bowl up to the deity candle and express your gratitude as you see fit. It's important here to speak from your heart: whatever words you say aloud will matter more if they're not rehearsed or provided by me.

Sit in your sacred space for as long as you like. When you feel comfortable, close the ritual in your usual way. Remember to take any excess energy back into yourself and ground as needed. Dispose of the milk and honey mixture outside if you are able, preferably in a garden or flowerpot.

As you move beyond treatment into survivorship, you'll hit anniversary after anniversary. The first year after I finished treatment, many of my anniversaries were painful: the anniversary of my diagnosis, my biopsies, my surgery, the first day of chemo, and the day I realized my partner was done with me. But there were also joyous "I beat cancer" anniversaries, like the day I finished chemo and smashed my porcelain bell, the first Thanksgiving and holiday season after treatment, the day I put a sparkly barrette in my newly grown white hair. I can tell you the pain of the bad anniversaries does fade with time, but the joy of the good ones doesn't seem to fade at all.

It's okay to be proud of your survival, and it's okay to talk about it. Celebrate those good anniversaries with something special, because cancer teaches us vital lessons about taking time for granted. Buy yourself flowers, take yourself out to dinner, get yourself celebratory presents, go on that trip with your partner and kids—you're all worth it, and why wait?

15

Living With Fear

About a month after radiation, I had my first meeting with the oncology nurse about what they call "survivorship." Because my breast cancer was "fed" by estrogen and progesterone, I was put on a hormone blocker, which I'll be taking daily until my body no longer makes those hormones. Hormone blockers reduce my risk of recurrence to under 10%, which is important because once you've had cancer, the risk of recurrence is never zero. That was a hard truth to accept and caused me enough anxiety and worry that I found a therapist that summer. The fear of recurrence was constant for me in that first year after treatment ended. Had I not gotten some help to heal the emotional and spiritual wounds after the ordeal on my body was over, I would've wasted opportunities to build a new life for myself.

If you don't have one already, I can't recommend finding a therapist after cancer treatment enough. Meditation, ritual, lighting candles, and doing spell work all help, but they are not a replacement for a mental health professional in the same way they are not a replacement for a medical team's treatment of your disease. You just spent quite a long while—since the average treatment plan lasts months at a minimum—fighting to stay alive and be as healthy as you can be. Why would you not invest the same time and energy into your mental health afterward? I've said before that cancer is a medical trauma, and you carry that trauma with you until you find a way to deal with it.

One of the hardest things about being Pagan is learning there is no magic that will get you out of doing the work yourself. Shadow work and processing what has happened is a spiral: you start at the surface and work a little on the easy thing, cry, journal, move on, and later something else comes up that brings you deeper, and you repeat the process. Therapy is hardcore shadow work with a guide who specializes in mental health. I had huge emotional responses and panics for a while every time I had a doctor's appointment, and was diagnosed with PTSD, depression, and anxiety after an exhaustive intake discussion.

My first mammogram after cancer was routine and gentle and over in all of ten minutes, but I barely made it out the clinic doors before I started crying. I sat in my car in the clinic lot ugly crying and frozen, unable to even see, for over thirty minutes.

The thing about panic attacks is they aren't reasonable. They are a fight-or-flight response that triggers overwhelming terror, feelings of helplessness, despair, anger, and a whole host of other icky feelings. Physiological responses include crying, hyperventilating, tightness in your chest, nausea, sweating, chills, elevated heart rate, and muscle clenching (as an example, my jaw and shoulders tighten up, which makes my whole upper back and neck clench). If your panic response is extreme or debilitating (or even if it's just annoying), please seek assistance. Really, there is *no* shame in getting help for your involuntary reactions. Your body, mind, and spirit have been through the wringer, and you don't have to do this alone, even after active treatment is over. Survivorship is another stage of cancer treatment, and the adjustment can be a struggle. You've practiced accepting a healthy amount of help all through your journey into this new reality, so don't stop now.

I am not a mental health professional, but I can tell you what has been working for me to try to mitigate these attacks. First, I spent a lot of time going over what my triggers are with my therapist so I can avoid them during dangerous moments (like while I'm driving or cooking) and start working through the feelings in a safer space. Make no mistake: processing these feelings is hard work, so it's okay to approach it in small chunks and take breaks in between. My personal triggers are getting a mammogram, having an IV inserted, and throwing up. These aren't really triggers I could do any sort of exposure therapy for (repeating the instance and try to wear down my emotional response), so I spend a lot of time thinking about them, writing about them, and talking with my therapist about them in hopes I can give my emotions enough of an outlet that I don't panic.

It's been a few years now since I finished treatment, and I still cry after I get a mammogram. It's not the sort of incapacitating terror it was that first time, but the reaction is still there. It is getting better with time, and that's the most awful thing to tell you. Time is a necessary ingredient to this work, and I don't know a way around it (please let me know if you find a way to speed this along).

I had help prioritizing which symptoms to handle and in what order because the maelstrom of panic makes everything such a swirling mess it's hard to see what helps the most from within. With my therapist's help, I worked on breath first, because feeling like I can't breathe makes me feel out of control.

EXPANDED BREATH WORK

Close your eyes and focus on breathing as deeply as you can. Focus *only* on your breath, because the panic response in your body is forcing you to breathe shallow and fast, which becomes a spiral that makes panic worse. Remember the five-five-five technique early in this book? That is *so* useful when you're trying to regain control. If possible, do this to a ten-count.

Sit up straight, like you have a string coming out from the top of your spine that you pull to make your upper body tall. This leaves room for your lungs to expand. It might take a few breaths to be able to do this, because for some of us, all those core muscles clench up and leave us hunched over. That's okay; just keep trying.

Breathe in and count to ten. Go ahead and breathe through your mouth if your nose is stuffy. Feel your diaphragm expand and relax your belly muscles if you can. Fill your lungs into your upper chest and your belly.

When you can't fit any more air in, hold your breath to the count of five to ten (whatever you can manage). Feel your belly and chest muscles release a little bit with the pressure of full lungs.

Release your breath through your mouth to a count of ten. That means releasing it slowly, and, as your chest and diaphragm relax, letting some of the tension in your neck and shoulders release.

Repeat this process at least five times, because it may take a few tries to get your body to respond and take in that full breath.

Deep breathing into your belly stimulates the vagus nerve, or the tenth cranial nerve. The vagus nerve is the longest nerve in the autonomic nervous system, so it affects the heart, lungs, and digestive tract (your "gut"). Essentially, it's part of what tells your body that you are in fight-or-flight mode instead of normal mode. If your breathing is shallow and fast, the vagus nerve tells your body you can't relax, you might have to run *right now*. If your breathing is deep and slow, you're telling your body the danger has passed and it's okay to resume normal processing. If you are a person who feels nauseated as a stress or panic response, deep breathing will tell your body it's okay to digest normally, you don't have to get rid of your food in preparation to run.

Once your breathing is under some control, keep your eyes closed and start focusing on unclenching your muscles. Roll your shoulders up, back, and down to let some of the tension out. Unclench your fists. Open your mouth wide to stretch your jaw and unstick your tongue from the roof of your mouth. If you hold tension elsewhere when you're wound up, like your lower back or legs, focus on relaxing those, too.

I find it useful to chant something simple and to the point:

> *"This will not control me. I am in no danger.*
> *I am in control."*

When you are able, ground yourself for a few moments, and let residual panicked energy drain as much as you can. Once your breathing is normal and you no longer feel like you're going to explode, drink a little water and maybe eat something. Panic attacks burn massive amounts of energy, so it's normal to feel depleted and exhausted after you've calmed down.

Other ways to combat a panic attack:

- **Naps:** As my friend and fellow witch Sarah says, never underestimate the power of a good nap.
- **Drugs:** Sometimes, an anti-anxiety medication is needed. This isn't a weakness or anything shameful,

it's just medication for an illness. If your attacks are debilitating and your therapist and doctors recommend extra help, don't be afraid to take that offer of assistance.

FOCUS ON FIVE SENSES EXERCISE

This exercise is intended to bring your mind's attention from the internal spiral of terror to the external reality around you. Sit or lie down in a space that is safe enough for you to close your eyes for a few moments. Close your eyes. Take three slow, deep breaths, then focus your attention on the following questions.

- What are you touching right now? Does it feel warm, cold, soft, hard, bumpy, comfortable, fuzzy, scaly?
- What do you hear? Describe it to yourself.
- What do you see if you can open your eyes (even if they're tearful)? Bright light? Darkness? What color do you see first? What objects are in your line of sight?
- What do you smell right now? This one might be tough if you've been crying, but it's still worth a try.
- What do you taste right now? Is there a copper taste of fear on the back of your tongue? Lingering flavors from the last thing you ate or drank (coffee aftertaste, maybe)?

Focusing your mind on what's tangible in the moment will help your body realize it's not in immediate danger, which may help you come out of the attack.

None of these suggestions will happen instantly. Panic isn't a mode you can switch off, but practice will allow you to recover faster and maybe ease the intensity of the attacks.

16

Ongoing Treatments

While active treatment is over when your surgeries, chemotherapy/immunotherapy, and radiation are finished, "cancer-free" doesn't mean "done with cancer." Survivorship looks like a lot of doctor's appointments, and not just with oncology. My annual mammogram was set, but my doctor wanted me to get new baseline medical stats on record, which meant getting a physical with my general practitioner, having an annual exam with my gynecologist, and seeing my dentist. Dentistry is put on hold during chemotherapy, even standard cleanings, because if bacteria is introduced while your immunity is low, an infection could start. During treatment, everything was about mitigating risk. In survivorship, everything is about prevention: not only preventing cancer recurrence but preventing any health issue with regular maintenance.

As a person with a medical history of cancer, my experiences at the doctor's and dentist's offices were markedly different from before the cancer. As an example, I have a lump on my right leg that no one worried about until after I was done with chemo and radiation. Though I'd had it for years, suddenly it needed X-rays and ultimately an MRI to confirm it wasn't serious (it was not). I was able to get COVID-19 vaccines and boosters right away, and I've had the pneumonia vaccine usually reserved for the elderly and immunocompromised. While I generally feel fine, I am reminded by my GP that as long as I'm on hormone suppression medication, I'm still in treatment.

Unfortunately, I also had to start my colonoscopy screenings earlier than most. It's not fun, it triggers me (the prep makes me vomit), and I hate it. But it's preventative maintenance that will help head off any cancer at the pass, so I do it annually. This is despite my genetic testing, which returned negative for the breast cancer genes, the colon cancer gene, and a few others. Genetically, there's no reason why I got breast cancer. But this is why sticking with checkups and tests is important, even in survivorship.

I think the most difficult part of the ongoing treatments is the slow recovery of physical and mental well-being after chemotherapy and radiation. I struggled with exhaustion and anemia post-treatment for well over a year. I manage it now with regular supplements and exercise, but sometimes it still just hits me in a wave and I nap or go to bed early.

I also still struggle with neuropathy (nerve damage) in my feet and "chemo brain." The neuropathy manifests in occasional numbness in the balls of my feet and my middle toes, and, more annoyingly, as a sudden violently strong itchiness on the bottom of my foot that can't be relieved. For some reason, that only happens when I'm driving long distances (therefore, I have shoes on and can't possibly do anything about the itch). Frustratingly, there's nothing to be done about the neuropathy except wait and see if the nerves heal themselves over time.

Chemo brain, which looks like forgetting words and events, forgetting names, inability to focus, and a general fuzzy feeling that makes thinking difficult, is the scariest of my long-term treatment side effects. It's so difficult to tell whether it's a normal brain lapse or something more serious, and as a writer, it's worrisome to lose words. It's been a few years now since I finished chemo, and while it did get better, my brain hasn't fully restored to BC functionality. I still lose words. I still have occasional brain blips on things like names or phone numbers I've known for a long time. Sometimes it's hard to remember appointments, addresses, and new acquaintances' details. It's frustrating and scary. Puzzles like word searches, sudoku, and crosswords were prescribed by my oncologist to help restore and maintain my brainpan.

Physical strength, endurance, and balance are also all slow to replenish. Be kind to yourself: if you were a marathon runner in top shape before cancer, even you will likely need time to rebuild. Vitality does return, and the small gains made in a week will compound as the year rolls on. This is your only meat suit in this lifetime. Treat it with love and respect and all the self-care rituals you've used before and during cancer. It may look and feel different, but it's still you. It's part of the new you that you create in survivorship for the rest of your life.

DAILY CHECK-IN RITUAL

Materials:
- A candle (choose its color based on what you'd like to focus on: blue for emotions, purple for spirit, green for physical health, or plain beeswax for all)
- A piece of jet or hematite, for purifying and grounding
- A journal
- A writing utensil

This can be done as a quick meditation to start or end your day, or a full ritual taking all the time you'd like.

Ground and center, and if you're doing a full ritual, perform your usual opening steps.

Light the candle, inviting your Deity if you wish for Their attendance.

Hold the stone in your hands and focus on the candle flame. Take three deep breaths and let the outside world fall away.

Close your eyes and do a scan of your body. Notice anything that stands out to you at this moment: are you hungry? Tired? Cold? Do you have numbness anywhere, or aches? Take a deep breath and hold it for a few seconds, then release the breath and allow your muscles to relax. Scan internally again and notice anything new.

Focus your attention on your emotions and mental state. What feelings are passing through you? What feelings would you like to let go of for the rest of your day? How is your mental clarity and focus today? Do you feel on top of things, or are you noticing a fuzziness around the edges? How motivated are you feeling at this moment?

When you're ready, set the stone down next to the candle and write down your impressions. It doesn't have to be a full journal entry: if you create a daily habit of jotting down quick notes for this ritual, you'll be able to pick out patterns later, particularly if you're tracking other things like diet, exercise, or hormonal cycles.

If it helps you focus, set your intention for the rest of your day (or the next day, if you do this at bedtime). Blow out the candle, close your ritual and circle if you opened one, and go on with your day.

This sort of mindfulness shouldn't be looked at as a big event in your day, but more as a healthy self-care habit to continue your wellness journey post-treatment. It's useful to help identify trouble areas as early as possible, and, with time, it's interesting to look back at the ways you've actively created a foundation of meaning for your new life.

17

THE NEW NORMAL

You deserve to be happy and have a full life after cancer.

That's it. No qualifiers, no justifications.

Okay, but how do you get there? How do you create a meaningful normal that makes you happy and fulfilled after going through hell for a year? I think, as Pagans, we're uniquely equipped with the tools to create a meaningful AC life in ways that others may not be, because we already create our own ethics, values, and meaning in our spiritual life. We are used to working for it, aren't we? Creating our own meaning means we have unlimited freedom in defining what makes our lives successful, purposeful, and valuable for ourselves. That's a double-edged sword because it's incredibly hard work to have that much freedom: it's easier to follow an established set of rules or values, to find someone who can tell you what to do or what to care about. It is my hope that you can use the Sabbat sections in the appendix as a jumping-off point to create your own meaning during your cancer journey because, while it is true that no one can do it for you, it is also true that no one can do it as well as you.

If, like me, you sort of floated through your life before cancer, creating a new life after cancer will be full of pitfalls and false starts. I was lost, and I alternately felt like crying and giving up or in a rush to do everything I couldn't during treatment. Of course, we were still in the first summer of the pandemic, so "everything" was heavily restricted anyway. I went to my family's cabin for a week to relax, read, swim, and try not to sunburn my barely covered noggin. I went to a trainer at the gym and told her what my last year had been like, how tired I was of being weak and tired, and that I needed to figure out how to fuel my body like a well-run machine instead of feeding it all the junk I'd been eating for the last forty-odd years. I started a whole workout and diet routine, motivated to never have to do chemo again.

Identifying what you'd like to add, change, or remove from your life is the easiest part. Following through takes time and consistency, which means it needs a plan. Plans for change don't have to be stressful or complicated, and you don't have to do this alone. Therapists, doctors, gym staff, teachers, friends, apps, websites: support comes in so many forms to choose from, so you can pick which works best for the next step in your journey.

Take the time to consider changes you've made to your spiritual routines while you were in treatment. Did you meet any new deities who helped you? Will you continue to build those relationships, or did you thank them and let them go?

Will you incorporate new, pared down techniques for your practice that you needed during treatment? Will you focus on strengthening and deepening your practice, or did you find you needed Paganism and witchcraft less during and after cancer? Both are legitimate positions.

Take stock of your finances and your financial planning post-cancer. What do you need to feel secure financially again? What do you need to feel fulfilled professionally? Are you happy in your current job, or did cancer give you a kick in the pants to do something else and make changes that are good for your long-term well-being? What's the state of your income and debts after cancer? Financial wellness is closely tied to mental wellness, and it's far better to have a clear picture of your status so you can make plans: actions to take that will bring you into a better position financially. This includes a debt-repayment budget, but it also includes saving for retirement and estate planning. I discovered last summer that I can't get life insurance until I'm five years cancer-free (which means five years after I ended chemo and radiation). It triggered some fear of recurrence, but it also had me write a big reminder on my calendar for my five-year anniversary.

Plans matter. Plans tell the universe you will be here, that you will be living your second life with intention and, dare I say, gusto.

A common theme I've encountered when talking about post-cancer mental health in survivorship is the total lack of tolerance for bullshit. Suddenly all those red flags in your job and unhealthy relationships that you've brushed off become untenable. The dreams you've been putting off for months, years, or decades, are all up for review, either to discard in favor of new dreams or to focus your energy on chasing, because time is a valuable loss when you've had cancer. The idea that you can do something later is always met with a quick follow-up thought that you may *not* have time, because our mortality and the uncertainty of this life is brought into sharp focus during chemotherapy and radiation.

Become aware of your own cycles in survivorship is essential, including spiritual cycles. Spirituality and witchcraft are what you make them, and meaning is created with intention. You move into a new life having faced a crucible of heavy physical, emotional, mental, and spiritual trials. Recovery and building a new life after cancer takes time, but it can be freeing, because you have a different perspective on the unpredictability of life and the preciousness of time. Do what brings you fulfillment in this lifetime. Be picky with your energy and attention: put it into whomever and whatever matters to you the most. *Live* your life.

While you're creating this new reality, fear and doubt will inevitably seep in. That's just part of the world and part of being human. When fears and doubts creep into my plans, I try to remember that positive affirmations work. Because words are spells, they work best when you say them out loud (although you can write them down in a daily journal as well). I've included a list I use regularly, but I suspect you have your own based on your revised priorities.

- "I am worthy of this life."
- "I am worthy of my loved ones."
- "I deserve to be happy, healthy, and whole."
- "I deserve to find success that suits me."
- "I deserve to meet my needs and pursue my wants."
- "I deserve to be treated with love and kindness."
- "I have lived through traumas, but they do not define my future."
- "I define my future."
- "I deserve to love and be loved."

That last one was particularly difficult for me, and due to my past, was difficult even before the extra weight of surviving cancer. For a time after I finished treatment, I thought having had breast cancer at all would somehow taint me from future romantic relationships. I kept thinking, "who on earth would want to date such a bad bet? I can't give anyone children, I can't make long-term plans, and I can't even promise I won't get cancer again because I do have some risk of recurrence." The deeply injured part of my heart thought it wasn't worth the time or effort to build a romantic relationship with anyone, because if my last partner left when he thought I'd die during treatment, I had to assume anyone else would do the same. Fuck the idea of opening myself up to that sort of pain again.

This is where my therapist's no-nonsense attitude was her greatest gift to me. As I worked through these fears while we talked of the man who left, she called a very sharp and firm bullshit on my woeful feelings. Instead of seeing what was out there, I was determined to fail before anything even started, an attitude that might well have been the end of me if I'd just given up when I was diagnosed and not bothered with treatment. She convinced me to experiment with an online dating app not to find love, but to prove to me that breast cancer survivorship wouldn't automatically disqualify me from the game. We set up my profile with "breast cancer survivor" as the first sentence. That way, if anyone expressed interest, I could assume cancer wasn't a deal-breaker, because they would've seen it before contacting me, and if it was, I'd never know.

Online dating in my forties after a divorce and then the breakup of my post-divorce relationship during cancer was a book of weird experiences all on its own, but ultimately, I did meet a man. He not only wasn't concerned I'd had breast cancer, but he also convinced me through both action and words that he is kind, stable, and honorable. I know all the way to my bones that he would never abandon me if I had another health scare. Not only did this man invite me into his life and support mine, but he also gave me what I thought I'd lost forever when I was diagnosed. He's a package deal, you see, and so when I married him, I became stepmom (or in our household, a bonus mom) to four excellent teenagers. I have told them more than once that this outcome was a lottery win for me, and something I could never have expected or predicted after a year of treatment. I think if I hadn't had therapy, I might've let this incredible opportunity for happiness pass, and that would've been a terrible side effect of cancer.

Survivorship is a new start. It likely looks very different from your life before cancer, but it is still your life, and you deserve this chance to build something new and meaningful and to find happiness.

My sincerest wish for you, if you'll allow me to wish for you, is the easiest treatment possible, as low a risk of recurrence possible, and a swift recovery of your vitality and power. You can do this.

APPENDIX

Celebrating the Wheel

SAMHAIN

I was diagnosed just before Samhain, which is my favorite of the sabbats. Admittedly, I've always been a bit lackadaisical about celebrating holidays, even after dedicating myself to the Morrigan. But my treatment followed the Wheel of the Year in a way that made each holiday more meaningful to me than all my years of more casual observances, particularly when my journey into darkness began just as I was preparing for Samhain. There is a perfectly reasonable explanation for the timing: October is Breast Cancer Awareness month in the US. A mammogram resulting in an anomaly required an ultrasound, which became a biopsy, which prompted an MRI, and bloop: I had a cancer diagnosis in the season of the dead.

A year-and-a-day is a standard measurement of spiritual work in Wicca and other Pagan groups: the time from declaration to initiation, the traditional length of a handfasting, and the time it takes to break a spiritual connection. So, while there was a coincidental explanation for my diagnosis just before Samhain, I found meaning and a message from Her in the timing. The turn of the wheel, beginning with Samhain, would be dedicated to beating cancer and learning how to build a new life in survivorship.

I am (to no one's surprise, I'm sure) an introvert, and I live in a state that tends to celebrate the warmer seasons with a desperate frenzy of activity. Samhain not only includes all the fun of Halloween traditions with my stepchildren, niece, and nephews, but it's also my signal that it's okay to slow down a little, rest, and revert my focus inward as the seasons change from the warmth and long light of summer to the icy darkness of winter. For the last twenty years or so, as I learned more of the Morrigan's lore and listened more to Her in my meditations, I've been called most strongly to Her service during Samhain. This book is written in service to Her after my first Samhain ritual post-treatment, where the idea presented itself with gusto and turned up in every Tarot reading, meditation session, and ritual for months after. The message couldn't have been clearer: support others in service to Her the way She supported me throughout my cancer journey.

There are multiple excellent resources on the Morrigan, and since She is not the specific topic of this book, I will gladly refer you to additional sources in the bibliography for further study. In my own practice and experience, my strongest connection to the Morrigan begins at Samhain. I spend a lot of time hiking or sitting in the woods in the late fall, talking to Her and meditating to listen for Her wisdom. That fall when I was diagnosed, I spent hours in my backyard at night or hiking in a local park at dusk, listening and praying. I've included a couple of my oft-used prayers below.

A Prayer to the Morrigan

*"Morrigan, Morrigan, Morrigan
Battle Crow, Phantom Queen, Washer at the Ford
Great Queen, help me do what needs be done.
I seek a guide as I step into the dark.
I seek your wise counsel as my battle begins.
Morrigan, Morrigan, Morrigan,
I ask you to walk with me, so I do not fight alone."*

A Prayer to the Lord and Lady

*"Lord and Lady, I am humbled by my illness.
Lord and Lady, I ask for your blessing.
Bless me with the gift of your guidance,
Help me face my fears with courage and grace,
Show me a way through these trials that I may walk
this path with dignity,
And honor you with my fortitude."*

There is no necessity to work with a particular deity during any celebration of the wheel, or any deity at all. Many friends of mine use Lord and Lady, the Universe, or another general term for what they think of as a higher power. Since Samhain is a liminal time where the veil between this life and the afterlife is thin, you can also speak with your ancestors instead of a deity if that works best for you.

Celebrating Sabbats has always been a private solace for me, and I was completely devastated by my diagnosis just weeks before Samhain. I wasn't excited for the family Halloween doings (for a few years, I decorated the basement of my house for my niece and nephews. It was as haunted and scary as it could be for kids under ten years old) or for my own private Samhain traditions.

Instead of a formal ritual that year, I set an extra place at the table when I ate dinner and thanked my ancestors. I lived alone at the time, so it was easy to chat with them out loud. My heritage is quite Scandinavian (I come by stubborn stoicism honestly), so I lit a candle to my Viking ancestors and thought for a long time that evening about the journey I was about to embark upon. Cancer treatment would be my combination of self-defense and exploration in hope for a better future. I was determined to face my enemy with honor, unflinching with the will to endure and prevail. I can't say the ritual took away my fears or gave me reassurance, because in my experience that level of certainty isn't possible. But it did help bolster me for the events to come, and for that, I'm grateful to my Norse heritage.

A Ritual to Honor Ancestors and Accept Help

Materials:
- Place setting (dishes, silverware, glass)
- Candle
- Ritual supper or food (whatever you're eating to celebrate)
- A bell (optional)
- Music (optional)
- Incense (optional)

If you use a more formal setting, start your music, light your incense, and cast your circle. Set a place at your table for your ancestors, including a chair. Light a candle in front of their setting.

If you have a bell, ring it, and say:

> *"Ancestors, I invite you to my table this Samhain, while the veil is thin, to join my dinner celebration."*

Dish a portion of the same food you are eating on the plate as if they're there, and say:

> *"Ancestors, I offer you this food in gratitude for your wisdom."*

As you eat your food, tell them what's on your mind, what fears you have going into treatment, or whatever else is on your mind. Ask them if they have advice or assistance to offer. Listen for responses, but know that response could come in feelings of being supported or in moments of strength later. You are asking, not demanding, and they are not obligated to respond.

When your dinner is over and you're ready to close, thank your Ancestors for attending. Tell them you'll be listening if they have advice or wisdom to share later. Then blow out your candle and take down your circle (if you cast one). Finally, whatever food on the extra plate can be composted, left outside for animals (if appropriate), or thrown away. If you keep an altar to your Ancestors in your house, appropriate food could be left there for the night, if it's safe to do so.

However you decide to celebrate Samhain, remember that, as the year's cycle descends into the darkest time, it is also a time of remembrance, rest, and renewal. In some traditions Samhain is the New Year, so just taking some time to look back on the past year's events and see how far you've come is a worthwhile exercise to celebrate the day in liminal space.

YULE

Prior to chemotherapy, I often celebrated Yule by sitting vigil until the sun came up, an exercise in faith that during the longest night, the light would return. Around my usual bedtime, I'd make mulled cider in a crock pot, a meat and cheese board (called a "shark-coochie" board in my house, a deliberate mispronunciation of *charcuterie*), and turn off all electronics and lights except the strings of twinkling holiday lights. The summer before I got cancer, I'd moved into a house with a wood burning fireplace, and I was so excited to be able to sit vigil until sunrise with my usual snacks, candles, lights, and a real fire.

Yule in 2019 fell on the Saturday after my first infusion. I'd spent that whole week feeling unexpectedly good. I was fighting a cold and had a bad cough (unrelated to chemo; an accidental gift from my partner) but overall felt okay, considering I'd willingly been poisoned. It was the first round, so I didn't know that the worst side effects hit after all the steroids and anti-nausea medications wore off.

I was getting in the ritual shower for the evening when dizziness and nausea hit hard, and I threw up. Not the ritual I intended. Instead of Yule fun, I spent the next few hours alternating between throwing up and fitfully dozing. I had to call my parents for help because I couldn't get down the stairs to let my dog, Ragnar, out. They spent a couple hours with him, made me drink water, and cleaned my bathroom. Not a shining moment in my adulthood, lying in bed in my forties watching my mom cleaning up my shower in the bathroom less than ten feet from my bed because my body was suddenly so weak and sick.

When the retching finally paused, I spent time lying under the warm covers meditating about death and rebirth. I couldn't burn incense due to my cough and nausea. There is a safe place on my altar to leave a candle burning for a while, so I lit it, quietly invited the Morrigan, asked Her to protect me while I fought this new battle, and went back to bed.

That's it. That was the only bit of my planned Yule ritual and vigil I was able to do that year. I woke at sunrise not on purpose, but because I'd slept hard enough to ignore any bladder needs until it was light. But I did greet the day and thank Her for the restful night before going back to bed, where I stayed for another couple of days.

In my experience, the gods are not looking for us to overextend ourselves to our detriment as an offering. It's okay to give yourself the time to heal, which is especially important during chemotherapy and radiation. If you're upset about missing your usual Yule observances or need to keep some sense of normality after your life has been punted into an abyss, set an alarm to wake up with the sun on the morning after the longest night. Greet the return of the light with long, deep breaths, and feel the energy of renewal seep into you (particularly if you live in the far northern hemisphere, where the light of winter is weak and the air can be powerfully cold). If you need to go back to bed afterward, do. Take care of yourself. Be gentle.

Ever since cancer treatment, I've dedicated my Yule celebrations to both the Morrigan and Persephone, who is simultaneously the Goddess of spring and the Underworld. That Yule, during the first real restful night's sleep I'd gotten that week, I dreamed of Persephone, and began including pomegranates and dedications to Her in my longest night ritual.

Interestingly, pomegranates are high in antioxidants, high in vitamin C, and have a strong flavor. I drank a lot of pomegranate juice that winter, and I include it as my ritual drink now for Yule because it's delicious, good for me, and I can pour some as libation to Persephone. Plus, it's a deliciously deep garnet red that insists on bringing the vibrancy of lifeblood to the colorless winter.

Persephone's story reminds me that the journey into darkness isn't permanent. The darkness is a time for rest and healing, and it can take a long time to recover from physical and emotional ills in our lives. Her eventual return to the light is a reminder that hope isn't dead.

I've included a guided meditation on Persephone below. If you have someone in your life whose voice you find soothing or uplifting, ask them to record reading it aloud so you can listen at your leisure. Or ask them to read it to you like a bedtime story while you sit or lie with your eyes closed. You can also read it aloud to yourself and record it or memorize it and go through the steps in your head as you journey.

Guided Meditation: Persephone

Sit comfortably with your back straight (no slouching) and hands at rest on your lap or lie down with a light blanket over you and a pillow under your knees. Close your eyes. Take a few deep breaths to ground and center yourself (see the technique described in Chapter One).

Let your mind drift in the darkness behind your eyes for a few breaths. If a thought passes through the darkness with you, give it a wave and let it keep floating on by. Breathe deeply for a five count, filling your lungs and letting your diaphragm relax into your belly. Hold the breath for a four count, then release it slowly, emptying your lungs of all the air and tension your body is holding. Breathe in again and float in the darkness as you hold and exhale. Let your body relax. The darkness here is comforting, warm, and safe.

Notice a light in the distance. It is faint and blueish, like a star in the darkness. Let yourself float toward it. You are not in a hurry: float gently through the warm dark of your inner self until the light gets brighter, a beacon that you can reach in space. A silver path appears below your feet, leading to the light. You walk toward it and come to a brightly lit silver door. It's covered in ornate carvings of flowers and vines. You test the handle. It is unlocked, and the door swings open silently to a huge field of wildflowers in the sun.

You step through the door and feel the warmth of the sun on your skin, smell the flowers' gentle perfume on the breeze. Bees buzz happily somewhere out of sight. Take a few moments and look around. Sit on the grass and notice the rolling hills around you, the clouds skipping across the sky that leave shadows on the field. What color is the sky? What specific plants can you see near you? What specific animals? Are there trees in the distance? Mountains? Any bodies of water nearby you can hear or smell? What does the grass feel like against your skin?

A hole appears in the side of the hill at the edge of the field. It's large—easily large enough to walk into—and looks almost like a cave entrance. You walk toward it and a woman appears. She's lovely, with long, loose hair and a flower crown. She carries a pomegranate in one hand. Her expression is sad as She beckons you to follow with Her free hand, and She steps into the cave.

You follow Her into the hole. The edges of the cave are jagged against the grassy hill, uneven and sharp, with roots sticking out to trip you. It looks like the cave was a sudden and traumatic hole torn in the field. Notice the details of the edges as you take your first steps into the darkness. What does the floor feel like beneath your feet? Is it stone or dirt? It smooths out as you descend, and you reach out to touch the side of the tunnel. Notice the scent of the earth around you and the way the air cools as you walk. The pomegranate in Her hand glows enough for you to follow as She descends into the darkness. This is different from the darkness of the inner self. Here, the lack of light feels close and unnerving instead of comforting. You keep the glow in sight, so you aren't lost in the tunnel.

A chamber opens before you. You can feel the pressure change as you walk into the room, as though the oppressive closeness of the tunnel has been lifted. The air is cold and damp. Has the scent changed? Your footsteps echo on stone floor, but Her footsteps do not echo. In fact, you can't hear her steps at all, but the faint red glow in front of you bobs along in the dark, leading the way. You walk slowly for a long time. It is scary and unnerving, being so unable to see what's coming. You follow the dim light and trust there is a path forward: you just can't see it in the thick darkness.

The light leads you through an archway you only get an impression of as the light floats through the opening, then suddenly candles and a fire blaze in the room. For a moment, the cure is as awful as the dark and you can't see, but you let your eyes adjust. She sets the pomegranate on a table in the center of a cozy room. There are thick carpets on the floor, bookshelves along the walls, a fire merrily crackling in the hearth, and something cooking that smells amazing. The walls glitter with embedded jewels, adding rich color to the room. The couch and chairs are comfortably overstuffed in velvety jewel tones matching the sparkles on the walls.

She offers you a plate. You politely decline, remembering stories of how She was trapped in the Underworld for months at a time. She laughs, delighted, and invites you to sit with Her a while and rest.

Take the time to notice details in Persephone's living room. She may advise you on how to make the best of your situation, on how to be patient while your life feels like it's out of control and descending into the dark. Spend as much time resting in Her company as you need.

When you're ready to return to the light, thank Her for Her time and guidance. She picks up the pomegranate light and leaves Her chamber lights on so you can see a little better as you journey back through the dark chamber. You cannot see the top of the room and feel some awe at the vastness of the cold darkness around you, but Her light is true and leads you through the earth across the floor to the entrance of the tunnel. Here, She says farewell and says you need to return to the light on your own, and it's okay if it takes time.

Slowly, you climb the dirt and stone tunnel, keeping one hand on the cold dirt wall as you journey back toward the surface. After some time, a light appears in front of you at the top. You are nearly there, and this has been a hard and scary journey into the dark, but that light at the top is a beacon leading you back. You are tired: your body aches with the effort and your muscles burn, but you continue moving slowly toward the entrance until the warm field of flowers is again before you, and you step out of the Underworld into the sunlight.

It's okay to rest for a bit and let yourself recover some strength before going back to yourself. When you are ready, walk across the field to the door waiting for you. Turn the handle and cross the threshold, following the glittering path before you into your own self. You pull the door closed behind you, but the path remains, leading you into the comforting space of your own body and mind until you can feel your body around you, breathing deeply. You are grounded here, safely secure in your own internal space.

Breathe deeply in counts of five in, five hold, five out. Wiggle your fingers and toes. Move your arms and legs and know this body of yours is not lost in the dark. You are here, safe, and the light is returning. Notice the light behind your eyelids and, when you're ready, open your eyes.

Be sure to eat and drink something to help bring you fully back to yourself. Know that you can visit Her field again if you have the need to find hope and light on the worst days.

IMBOLC

Imbolc in Minnesota is a dark and cold time in the best years. February is generally our coldest month (below zero degrees Fahrenheit, the air hurts your face, and frostbite can happen in minutes), and though the days have started to lengthen, the sunlight is still weak. The sky is often grey and bleak, and everything looks washed out, like it's been overlaid with a color-sapping filter. Imbolc never feels like the beginning of spring to me, but I do think of it as the beginning of the year's work and reigniting the fires of inspiration and passion. If the time between Samhain and Yule is for rest and renewal, the time between Yule and Imbolc is for planning.

Imbolc is probably the easiest Sabbat to do with no energy, simply because it's meant to bring energy back into life. I was in the middle of chemo at the time and on long-term sick leave from work, so I spent many hours bundled up in bed or on the couch binge-watching *Hawaii 5-0* and dreaming of future vacations. All that time stuck in the house because treatment leaves you with no energy is perfect for planning.[3]

---

[3] A note about being stuck inside in winter for those of us in harsher climates. If you can, take a little walk outside every day, even when it's ridiculously cold and you don't feel like it. The cold can perk you up a bit: it gets your blood flowing, and if you do it every day, you will feel the changes coming in the seasons even if you don't have the energy to do your usual workout or outside routines. February is where I notice the sunlight lengthening by a few minutes a day: at Yule sunset is around 4:30 p.m. here, and by February, it's passing 5 p.m. It makes a notable difference to my mental health, seeing and feeling that light coming back every day. My oncology nurse suggested that just getting up to walk to the mailbox is useful when you're in treatment, and the longer you can be outside, the better it is for you.

Also, the very act of writing down a plan sends a serious positive "I will beat this" attitude into the Universe, so while you're trapped and immunocompromised, think about what you'll do when you feel better.

IMBOLC RITUAL I

Materials:
- A fancy notebook or blank journal
- A favorite writing utensil (I prefer the fancy gel pens, but anything will work)
- Art supplies, if you want to decorate the cover or pages
- A candle and your favorite incense if you can stand the smoke and scent (leave this off if it makes you feel ill)
- Frankincense, cedar, dragon's blood, or your favorite cleansing essential oil

A quick practical note: you can absolutely use the notepad on your bedside table, your phone's list or note app, or a laptop. The purpose of dedicated items is to help you switch from mundane mind to sacred space mind. Dedicating a new notebook or journal to this effort imbues it with your energy even when you have little. Physically writing down goals helps make them firm in your mind, and therefore firm in the Universe. Typing is also writing; do whatever works best for you.

There is always time to call the quarters and cast a circle, particularly the first time you use the materials. I didn't have much oomph for doing formal ritual each time I worked on plans, so after cleansing and dedicating, I just kept them near me on the couch and would jot down ideas between naps.

If you can tolerate a candle and incense, light them and take a moment to ground and center yourself. Bless yourself with the incense smoke. Cleanse the instruments by passing them, one at a time, through the flame and the incense smoke (carefully, and if you do decide to use a laptop, you may want to use the alternative cleansing below).

If you can't stomach incense or if you're unable to have a lit candle in your space, it's okay to skip this step. Instead, hold your items in your hands and close your eyes. Visualize the same soft blue-white light used in a ritual shower or bath and use it to surround the materials like a cleansing cloud. See it swirling around the items and your hands, the flow of light washing away any dark splotches or external energy. When the light is clean and settled, let it go and open your eyes.

Using a drop of your favorite oil on the tip of your right index finger, draw a symbol on the cover of the notebook or journal (or closed laptop) that you use to identify something as sacred to you. A lucky sigil, a spiral, a pentagram, a rune, or even a heart or star can be meaningful. If you don't have a symbol you use most often, try meditating for a bit in that sacred space and draw what pops into your mind. It could be a candle flame to symbolize your passions, or a tree to symbolize rebirth and potential: there is no right or wrong answer here.

Decorate the front of your notebook (the cover, inside cover, or even the first page) with the art materials. Your decorations can be as simple as a title or as fancy as an elaborate picture. Spend some time on this: the intent of this planner is for what you can do in the future, which means you're planning to *have* a future.

A note here about why I'm not saying a plan for when this is over: not all cancers go into remission, and not all are completely cured. Even with a Stage IV diagnosis, planning for your future is still important because hope and a sense of purpose matter when in the throes of treatment. It's worth the energy to invest in your future, since no one knows what will happen next.

So, now you have a sacred spot for your plans. What do you put in there? There are big-ticket events everyone wants to be around for: a child's dance recital, a wedding, holidays, graduations. Write them down, but also write down things you want to do or see when you have the energy again.

- Make a list of places you want to visit, whether they're local or international. Restaurants, museums, and the cabin in the summer all count!
- Is there a particular hobby you want to work on again? Art, writing, film, music?
- Is there a business you want to open?
- A sport you want to try?
- An anniversary, recovery, birthday, or wedding celebration you plan on hosting?
- Are you a gardener? This is a fabulous time to work on your garden plans for the upcoming season, which rolls into the second Imbolc ritual below.

This is your space, and there are no time constraints here. Write down what comes to mind, and then set it aside. Hold the ritual space open for as long as you like, meditate, or even nap a little, but remember to close it when you're finished. The journal is now yours for planning your next adventures. Eat a little something if you did a full ritual and drink some water. It's good for you.

Imbolc is traditionally about sowing seeds for the future and often coincides with lambing season in the British Isles. I often get my herb garden started at Imbolc, because even if planting season where I live doesn't come until late May, indoor herbs are good for many uses both magical and mundane. You could do the ritual below with the materials listed, or just as easily with one of those nifty Indoor Herb Garden kits, ordered online and delivered right to your door, no journeys outside needed. If you have animals in your house (like my cat fAngus, Destroyer of Greens, who made himself deathly ill chewing on leaves before I caught him and got rid of the offending plant), it's worth checking whether the herbs are pet friendly.

Imbolc Ritual II: Planting the Seeds

Materials:
- 3–6 small indoor plant pots
- Herb seeds of your choice: rosemary, thyme, basil, chives, catnip, and lemongrass are some good options
- Indoor potting soil from any garden or hardware store
- 1 cup milk (optional)
- 1 pitcher water

I've done this ritual at the kitchen table where I can sit down and take breaks as needed. Lay out your materials within easy reach so you don't have to get up. Have a little snack and a glass of water nearby for yourself.

Close your eyes and take a few moments to ground and center and focus your attention on intent. Sowing seeds is an investment in the season to come; sowing edible plants with your own hands is an investment in your future health.

Set your plant pots in a row on the table. Fill each pot to about one and a half inches below the top with potting soil. Using your finger, make a small hole (or if the pot is large, a few small holes) about one-half to three-quarter inches deep in the soil.

Hold each seed (or series of seeds, if you are planting more than one in a pot) in the palm of your hand. Cover your palm with your other hand and close your eyes. Feel energy from deep in the earth travel up through the floor into your feet through your body to your hands. Feel the dark space in your palms, where the seeds are getting warmer, imbued with energy.

If you have a prayer, spell, or wish to make, you can do that now. If not, visualize the potential plant in your hand bringing health and wellness to you as it grows. Drop the seeds in the appropriate pot's hole(s) and gently cover with soil. If you celebrate Imbolc as lambing season or include Deity in your Sabbats, you can make an offering with a few drops of milk in the pot at this time. Water gently but thoroughly. (You don't want to wash away the seeds.) Repeat this process with the rest of your seeds and pots and set them where they'll receive the best sunlight until spring arrives.

Every time you water your seeds, remember that this is an investment in your future as well as the garden's.

OSTARA/SPRING EQUINOX

The spring equinox is all about finding balance and patience. The light that stays longer and longer each day is now equally sharing the stage with the darkness. Warmth increases every time the sun makes an appearance. Green shoots poke through the dirt carefully, because in Minnesota, snow can still blanket fresh grass and tulips in March and April. The chaos of spring brings impatience and cabin fever to everyone. And if you're in the middle of your five months of chemo, like I was, spring and warm weather is infuriatingly slow to arrive.

I've never run a marathon. In junior high, I was a sprinter and a high jumper in track (I was good at neither), but I never had the patience for long distance running. Chemotherapy is a marathon, and it's important to remember that there's a delicate balance between feeling better and overdoing something when you're not ready.

By the equinox, I was two months into the easier weekly infusions of Taxol. Oncology promised it would be easier than the Red Devil and I'd start to feel a little more human again, and they were right. My hair started growing back in fine wispy white down on my head (eyebrows and eyelashes, sadly, were last to come back). I put a little weight back on because I could eat without getting sick, although my sense of taste was still wonky. I felt better. But I wasn't back to normal, and cancer reminds you quickly and mercilessly that you aren't fully healed, so you have to find a balance between doing more and resting. Amusingly, my comment on finding balance has a literal example.

From the start of treatment, my medical team stressed that I'd have more energy if I exercised while undergoing chemo, but for the first couple of months, I could barely get out of bed. I lost muscle mass and strength right along with forty pounds. I've been a physically strong person all my life, and took for granted that if I felt better, I must *be* better. I decided to do some yoga in my living room one day, thinking yoga would be a gentle way to get back into working out. Perhaps it would've been had I not started with sun salutations.

I was on my first downward dog pose when my legs gave out and I tipped over, landing in an ungraceful heap with shaking arm and leg muscles. It was an excellent reminder that my body is still working hard on healing, and maybe I shouldn't push.

My best recommendation to you in celebrating Ostara or the spring equinox is to find something that makes you feel balanced. If you've been bedbound and trapped inside for the winter due to weather and illness, get outside for a while. Start the long road of rebuilding energy with a walk and light weightlifting. There are so many apps out there for our various devices, and when you're as weak as I was, a couple cans of soup work great as weights. If you've been pushing hard lately and haven't taken time for yourself, do so. Read a book in the sun, take a nap, or cook something fresh that makes you think of spring. Spend time with a friend or family if you've been hibernating with treatment and winter keeping you away from others (although, please take appropriate precautions if you're immunocompromised). Whatever you do on Ostara should help you bring a little balance back into a life that has been focused on getting to the next infusion, mitigating the next time you'll be ill, or what news you'll get at the next doctor's appointment.

Ostara is also a fertility holiday, which means it sits on the cusp of new energies that will flow after the day of balance tips toward warmth and abundance. Coloring eggs is an easy, family-friendly way to celebrate and do some healing spells using both signs and color magic.

OSTARA EGG HEALING ENERGY SPELL

Materials:
- Hard boiled eggs (as many as you want to bespell)
- Egg dye or food coloring in various colors
- Wax crayons in various colors
- Glass or plastic cups with about ¾ cup of cold water in each (one for each dye color)
- Spoon or egg dipper for dyeing

Think of each egg the way you would a candle spell: the inside is full of potential and energy, and the outside is a blank canvas for your spell work. Choose your crayon and dye colors based on what you consider to be a healing color, not just for physical health but also for mental, spiritual, financial, and relational health. Balance includes all aspects of your life, and it's possible you've been paying so much attention to cancer that you could use a bump of good energy in other areas.

Mark the shells with runes or sigils for health and vitality before you dip your hard-boiled eggs in dye, using colors that represent wellness and healing for you. You can do any combination of signs and colors that feel right to you. Focus your intention as you write or draw on your eggs and remember to be patient while the dyeing process occurs. Experiment with your color and sign combinations: there is no right or wrong pattern here.

Eat one of your eggs after you've dyed it to ingest the full potential of that spell for wellness or vitality. The others that you want to eat can be kept in the fridge until they're gone. You can also keep one or two out on your altar for a few days over the holiday as an offering to your Deity, as well as a reminder to put your energy toward sustaining this marathon through the end.

I saw a fabulous new contraption in the toy department that holds a hard-boiled egg on a sort of mechanical spinner, and instead of dyeing the egg, you make color patterns with markers. This is utter genius and would work like a charm (pun intended) for a low-energy Ostara activity. It's also an excellent idea for the kids to do instead of the mess of dyeing if you want to share this ritual with your children.

Depending on how long you leave them, you won't want to eat any eggs left out on an altar (or hidden in the yard for kids to discover). I know that sounds like common sense, but it seems worth repeating because while your immune system is compromised, it's important to avoid bacterial and viral invasions wherever possible. If it's been a day or more, you will want to find a different disposal method for those eggs. If you have a yard or woods, you can break the shells and leave them for animals to eat. Or you can bury them whole in the garden as offerings to the gods.

If an egg activity is just too much effort during treatment, try one of these activities instead:

- Watch the sun rise and set (with naps in between, of course).
- Color, draw, or paint. The equinox is a springtime activity, and spring is all about creating new colors and vibrancy in the world. It doesn't matter if you have one of those fancy adult coloring books with intricate patterns, borrow one of your kids' books, do a paint-by-number (yes, they're back and available online), or if you just do your own work. Add a little color to your world somehow, even if it's only for a few minutes.
- Eat something fresh and light: lemonade, salad, fruits, vegetables, or whatever you can stomach during chemo. Pay attention to the taste, texture, and scents, and let yourself be in that moment.
- Get yourself some spring flowers (this is a great way for your kids or spouse to help you celebrate if you aren't feeling up to doing much) and recognize the beginning of a bountiful season.
- Meditate and have a chat with Persephone, who was (and remains) the Goddess of spring long before Queen of the Underworld on renewal and rebirth.
- Spend time outside if the weather permits. Sit in the sun on the deck with a blanket over your lap or take a walk. If you have energy, go to a park and check out how your local flora is waking up.

Ostara is a hopeful holiday, so I hope you find some balance that tips you from the terror and stress of cancer to a sense of peace, even if it's just for a moment.

BELTANE

I love Beltane (also *Bealltainn, Bealtaine, Beltaine,* or however you prefer to spell it). Beltane is a fertility holiday full of sexual energy, among other points of view: if you are in the right circumstances and feel well enough to do so, it's a positive burst of energy to have sex as part of your celebrations. Traditionally, Beltane was a celebration of lust and the joys of physical connection, so enjoy yourself or your partner(s) and celebrate whatever fun your body can manage.

However, your treatment may still have your libido in hibernation, and that is also perfectly okay: forcing yourself to do something sexual if you feel like crap is not just silly, but also self-harming behavior. Beltane should be about finding joy, not obligation (sexual or otherwise).

The fertility fire festival marking summer's beginning in the Celtic Pagan calendar has always been full of fun, flirtation, and promises for me, even when I'm not celebrating in any sort of romantic or sexual way. Beltane (in the northern hemisphere) draws out all the excitement of possibilities on the cusp of summer's coming abundance.

I had my last chemotherapy treatment three days after Beltane 2020. If you're a *Star Wars* fan, it was May the Fourth, and I was certain the force was with me that day. I was tired, relieved, and a little trepidatious about the next step, radiation, but deep down I felt like the worst was over, and therefore I was jubilant. My family and I were supposed to go to the beach that May for a week, which would've been my opportunity to celebrate the fertility of the coming season with a dip in the ocean (a favorite of mine), but in May 2020, the country was still mostly on lockdown and travel was ill-advised. So, we delayed the trip for a year, and I spent my saved-up vacation fun money on a backyard hammock instead—not the camping hammocks that hang from trees or the inexpensive sort that often come out in spring and summer at camping and sporting goods stores, oh no. I went all out and got a specialized hammock that fit up to eight hundred pounds because I wanted to leave room for a second person to cuddle on the hammock with me. It was a sign of hope. I intended to spend my time outside that summer as much as possible, and I counted the addition to my backyard a promise to my future self that I would make the most of every regained minute.

That's what I want you to consider when you find yourself celebrating Beltane while under cancer treatment. You may not be even close to done with treatment; you may be just beginning your journey, but the magic of this time of year can still be harnessed for you.

When I do any fire ritual for this holiday, I make sure it's about celebrating the joy of possibilities, not anything negative. How you speak to yourself is important in aligning your mind, body, and spirit, especially when dealing in spell work or cancer treatment. "Should-ing" all over yourself causes regrets and self-recrimination, and negative statements, like using "won't" or "not," can pull focus from what you want or need. Spell work is more effective when your mind, heart, and soul believe what you're saying. As you consider what to write and burn in the fire ritual below, keep in mind that positive statements are more powerful.

A note before the ritual: jumping the Beltane fire (which I suspect began as a way for young men to show off and catch the eye of their love interests) is a challenge I've historically avoided due to my severely underdeveloped grace. If you have the oomph and agility to tend a fire and jump it to signify a faithful and courageous leap into your next adventure, I'm impressed, and I say more power to you. I've occasionally been able to have two fires to walk between, but even that can be tricky depending on your available space and weather conditions. It's okay to leave the actual firewalking to others and just watch the flames.

If you don't have the energy to have a bonfire (or a small and perfectly respectable campfire in some sort of backyard, or driveway firepit) for the ritual below, you could use a candle in a bowl of water or sand. If you are bedbound or too ill to have a fire, skip that portion and just do the journaling and spell slips when you can. And, if you're lucky enough to have a wood burning fireplace in your house, use it!

Fire Ritual for Healing

Like with other celebrations, if Beltane is a particularly bad day for energy or illness, delay. I don't know any deity who wants you to over-exhaust yourself to the point of harm or depletion for a ritual, whether it's for them or for yourself.

Materials:
- Wood: I prefer birch and oak. Birch burns fast, hot, and clean, while oak burns slower, so you end up with a longer lasting fire that starts and stays burning easier than using oak alone.
- Firestarter: fatwood or a small fire starter work fabulously for both indoor and outdoor fires and are less fussy than newspaper, cardboard, or small sticks when you're low on patience and energy. I've also done this ritual with one of those fire logs you can get at the grocery store that burns for 3–4 hours.
- A large candle, set in the middle of a glass bowl filled at least halfway with sand or water. If you use a candle instead of a larger fire, set a cauldron or firesafe bowl next to it.
- Matches or a lighter

- Writing utensil
- Bay leaves or scraps of paper
- A healing herbs sachet that doesn't make you nauseated during chemo, or one tablespoon each of cinnamon, clove, ginger, and nutmeg, mixed in a folded paper envelope or a sachet bag
- Journal or notebook

Take a moment to touch your materials and ask for your Deity's blessing. If you have the oomph and wish to, call your guardians and invoke your circle. Create a circle large enough for you to move around the fire, if possible, but at least enough room to sit in front of the flames (or candle) with your writing setup.

Start the fire and invite your Deity to join you in this endeavor. Take some time to reflect on your goal for this ritual: general healing? More energy? Specific ailments? I did this when I still had numbness in my toes and wanted the feeling to return. Include your mental and emotional ailments in your considerations as well: are you battling depression? Loneliness? Despair?

Write down the specific physical, emotional, or mental requests on your bay leaves, but take care to write them in a way that you are bringing things to yourself. This is not a banishing fire, but a drawing and healing fire. If you need more energy, write: "Energy is abundant within me." If you are depressed or despairing, write what you want to happen on the bay leaves, such as "joy returns to me" or "hope lives within me." Take your time with this exercise: there is no limit to what healing you're asking for, nor is there a time requirement other than when your flames run out of fuel.

When you're ready, walk in a circle around the firepit three times clockwise. If you're using a candle, present your sachet of herbs to the fire in a circular motion three times.

Go slow if you're low on energy and walk close enough to feel the warmth of the flames. Let the fire's cleansing heat burn away the sickness around you.

On the first circle, say:

"Let the holy fire of Beltane cleanse me."

On the second circle, say:

"Let the holy fire of Beltane energize me."

On the third circle, say:

"Let the holy fire of Beltane heal me."

Throw your sachet of herbs or spices into the flames and take your place by your pile of written ailments. One by one, hold one of the bay leaves in your hands, close your eyes, and visualize pushing the sickness from you into the leaf, leaving room for what you want to draw toward you. Throw the leaf into the fire and let it burn completely before selecting the next leaf. Continue until your pile is gone.

Take the time to journal about what you asked to be healed and how you feel at the end of the ritual. There is no rush: enjoy the fire, earth, and outdoors as long as you can. Remember to thank any invited guardians and deities before closing your circle. Then, go eat something springlike and healthy to nourish your body and mind while healing.

If you are too ill to do anything for Beltane, have a lovely cup of tea and go outside in the sunshine for a few minutes, or open a window for a little while and let the wind blow refresh the air in your house. Fresh air is its own sort of healing balm, and if your cancer journey is anything like mine, you likely need some.

MIDSUMMER/LITHA

Litha, or Midsummer, is a fertility and abundance holiday, and seeds sown earlier in the year should be growing with gusto. If you're a gardener, I'm sure this is a wonderful holiday for you, and if you're a gardener in cancer treatment, I hope the frenzy of growth and sheer green aliveness of the season gives you energy and rejuvenation.

In my journey, the month leading to Midsummer was all about radiation therapy. I finished chemo in the beginning of May and was on the road to some level of recovery for a few weeks before I had to start twenty-four rounds of daily radiation. My hair was growing back in earnest, which was both exciting and weird. I had these baby hairs just poking through during the last month of chemo, which sprouted into stark white stubble. It was unnerving; my head became an albino chia pet with no eyebrows or eyelashes. I was also extra susceptible to sunburn, so nobody saw my not-completely-bald head outside without a hat.

I was outside all the time that summer. My basil plants exploded with growth. My rosemary and impatiens had filled out their pots with lovely scents and color. My cilantro grew so obnoxiously fast that I couldn't harvest it all before it went to seed. My little planter garden thrived that summer, and my sense of smell returned in time for the intoxicatingly strong scent of herbs to flood the back yard. I spent hours on the hammock staring up through the leaves of the bay laurel tree in my yard and throwing sticks for my dog, Ragnar, who was ecstatic that I could come out with him again.

I was off medical leave and working remotely, just getting back into the routine of an office job, when I started radiation. My appointments were a theoretically manageable half hour long on every business day, so they didn't directly interfere with my job. But they slowly and inexorably sapped my energy right back to chemotherapy levels.

The first week was easier than anything I'd done for cancer treatment. By the end of the second week, I was a little tired and my right armpit was just a little tender. I used recommended lotions and aloe vera often, as instructed, and drank a ton of water. It was okay. By the end of the third week, the fatigue was noticeable. By the last week, I was so tired that a simple chore like washing a load of laundry wore me out for the entire day. The cumulative effects of radiation were utterly exhausting, and no amount of protein, exercise, or caffeine helped.

I discovered the worst side effect about a week after my final appointment, when the actual burn appeared in my armpit. It hurt worse than any burn I've had in my life, and it seemed to work itself out from the inside, like a bruise that's so deep it doesn't appear for a few days and takes a long time to heal. It was an angry red and purple with open, oozing sores, like a terrible blistering sunburn you'd have checked by a doctor.

It took a little over a week for my armpit to heal, and I still have scars today. I will also need to be extra careful about sun exposure in the areas I received radiation for the rest of my life, because that skin is significantly more prone to burning.

For Midsummer, since I couldn't go swimming or expose my burns, and because I was so unbelievably exhausted, I focused all my celebration on relaxing outside, spreading out my little rituals over the course of the day.

I greeted the sun (something I generally avoid because, despite my desire to learn to be a morning person, 5 a.m. has always been untenable to me). Then I went back to bed. I did a little gardening in my yard and patio containers. I ate strawberries and yogurt (in place of cream) and fresh greens picked up at the local farmers market and felt thankful for the summer abundance. I spent time meditating, grounding, and centering, so I visualized the bounty of Midsummer's energy rising to replenish and heal me. I napped in the hammock that afternoon in the shade, while the dog played or napped on the grass underneath me. I made sure I was awake at sunset to watch the day gently drift into darkness. My active treatment was over, and the next day was the beginning of my second life.

LUGHNASADH/LAMMAS

In the Wiccan Wheel of the Year, Lammas commemorates the death of the grain god and celebrates the first harvest. Rituals for group participants often include some funerary rites honoring the pain involved in a sudden death or loss. Grieving is part of the procession of the ritual.

In Irish Paganism, Lughnasadh coincides with the death of the god Lugh, and historically includes the community gathering for a funeral feast and athletic games, matchmaking, settling legal disputes and implementing new laws, storytelling, and trading. It was also a time to honor and grieve for those lost to an unexpected death. Basically, Lughnasadh was *the* summer event for multiple families and tribes, because as the season wore on and harvesting activities became more urgent, journeying for a larger gathering was less ideal.

I'm not strictly Wiccan, but I appreciate the death/rebirth cycle of the overall Wheel, especially when Lammas coincided with the beginning of what oncology calls the "survivorship" phase of treatment. As the stress of active treatment ceded space in my mind, the grief I'd set aside in favor of focusing on survival forced its way into my attention. Survivorship is no joke.

Lughnasadh was also when I started doing full rituals again because I had enough energy to manage both the mental and physical payments. Since the holiday is the first harvest holiday of the season and is traditionally focused on grains, I baked. I made herbed white bread and shortbread cookies and zucchini bread and a blueberry galette. (I may have been overcompensating for my lack of energy in prior months.)

None of my recipes are my own, or I'd share them here. My favorite bread recipe is from the book *Artisan Bread in 5 Minutes a Day* by Jeff Hertzberg and Zoe Francois. My favorite shortbread cookie recipe came in the box of my shortbread pan. Zucchini bread and blueberry galette are both from *Betty Crocker* cookbooks. When I'm baking any recipe, the things I do to make it my own have more to do with the symbols, herbs, spices, or oils I include and the chants and energy I put into the mixing, kneading, and baking.

When kneading and shaping bread, I often add rosemary and thyme to the dough. Both are healing herbs, and both are beneficial to recovery of both mental and physical health from a magical perspective. Even now, years later, this is my favorite bread to make for the holiday and in general, particularly since the brain fog that comes with chemotherapy doesn't disappear when treatment is over. I'll take every little bit of help I can get to make my new normal the best it can be. I also add a little sea salt on the top of the loaf and carve a sigil in the top before baking. The sigil can be whatever symbol is meaningful, although due to some weirdly decorated errors, I do recommend not using a complex pattern.

When mixing batter for cookies or cake, I mix clockwise and pour good intentions into the bowl right along with the other ingredients like a good kitchen witch. I've used lavender sugar instead of plain when making shortbread, or a citrus peel like orange or lemon. I add cinnamon, cloves, and nutmeg to my pancake batter.

I make something with fruit every year for Lughnasadh, preferably blueberries or strawberries because they're local to my area and still in the tail-end of the season. Anything I make with those, from muffins to yogurt parfaits to pie, is included in my ritual offering to the gods along with a hunk of bread. If all the offering food is safe for animals, I leave the offerings outside after ritual. For me, Lughnasadh is about celebrating flour, fruits, and abundance, so anything I make that day is offered in some portion to the gods.

Okay, so what if you're not in a mood to bake? What if you can't stand the smell of baking because of where you are in treatment? What if you don't have the energy to do all the rigamarole involved in baking anything from scratch?

I've celebrated Lughnasadh by eating a piece of store-bought bread toasted with a smear of butter or jam (I prefer jam, but I have a terrible sweet tooth). I have left cookies baked from pre-mixed dough outside for birds and squirrels to eat. I've gone for a walk in the woods and tossed blueberries and birdseed around willy-nilly while asking for continued abundance and the favor of my gods. I've harvested herbs from my own garden and thanked both the plants and the gods for their gifts.

It's also important to mourn. Allow yourself the time and space to let some of your grief escape, whether it's in full ritual or not. If you feel good enough to walk, run, play a sport, hike, or swim, go do that in honor of those who cannot. If the heart of this holiday is to be grateful for the first harvest of the season and honor sacrifices made by those who left us too soon, then whatever you do will be enough if you mean it with sincerity.

MABON

Mabon, the fall equinox, is the last day in the season before the amount of darkness overtakes the amount of light. It's the opposite balance from Ostara, celebrating the harvest and preparation for hunkering down for winter. From a Wheel of the Year perspective, this is the big harvest abundance holiday: decorate the altar with representation of the summer's-end bounty and make offerings of gratitude to the gods. As daylight recedes for the upcoming cycle, Mabon is a good time to review what doesn't serve you any longer and identify places you could be more balanced in your life.

By the time Mabon rolled around, my sense of taste was fully back (yay!), which means I was putting weight back on. I joyfully participated in the seasonal abundance of pumpkin spice everything and had gotten into a habit during chemo of eating whatever I could keep down (even if it was unhealthy). That habit was necessary when medication made it hard to eat, but it became unhealthy as my body stopped rejecting food. I'd lost any semblance of balance after treatment, and ongoing cancer recovery is supposed to include eating and exercising in more healthy ways. I was working out regularly with my new trainer, so I was developing better movement habits, but I was still unbalanced with eating. Obesity is something I've struggled with for most of my life, but now it is a risk factor for cancer recurrence.

I was also unbalanced in my mental health. Grief and fear had overtaken my mental state after Lughnasadh because there was just too much to process alone. I found a therapist and worked hard that fall at resolving issues around love and partnership, fear of recurrence, and medical post-traumatic stress.

Finding balance can be extremely practically difficult and emotionally taxing. In both of my examples, it turned out I needed to discover and name the issues, identify possible solutions, and recognize that letting them go would take time and consistency. Writing down your issues on a bay leaf and throwing it into the fire to be removed is a great first step, but that's just the beginning. All change takes time and consistent effort.

Your Mabon ritual can certainly be a mirror of your Ostara ritual with fire and bay leaves, if you change your intent to drawing out what no longer serves you and asking the fire to burn it away. There is an element of grace, forgiveness, and gratitude to letting things go. When we hold onto something unhealthy, it's far too easy to blame ourselves for waiting too long, allowing behaviors that are harmful, or condemning ourselves with shame. But none of that brings balance or peace, and it tightens the grip on things you're trying to release. Try to recognize that whatever unhealthy habit or feeling you want to release was with you for a reason, and let it go with gratitude if you can (that's not a prescription: there is some heavy stuff to handle with cancer, and not all of it is anything to be grateful for).

My post-traumatic stress and anxiety was trying to protect me from additional harm and fear. I'm neither weak nor a failure for that. My unhealthy eating was a response to chemo attempting to starve me, and my survivorship attitude of "this is my second chance and I'm going to live fully without restriction." These are completely understandable responses, but not sustainable long-term if I want to maintain my health. My fear of any romantic attachment was a protective reaction to what happened with my significant other during cancer, but it would hold me back from potential future happiness if I held onto it, and that wouldn't be any sort of balance.

Mabon Exercise in Identifying Imbalance

Materials:
- Journal or notebook
- Writing utensil
- White or beeswax candle in a holder or bowl
- Lighter or matches
- Flat space for writing (I do this at a table)

Set your candle in the holder or bowl in the center of your flat space and light it. Create your sacred space and set your circle. If you have deity relationships, asking for guidance or insight is appropriate. I didn't include incense in this meditation, but if you have a favorite blend that sets your mind and mood in a sacred space, please include it.

The journal or notebook and writing utensil should be close enough to grab from a seated position. Ground and center yourself and breathe deeply for a few minutes, settling into your position and body. Sink into the darkness behind your closed eyes and absorb any messages your mind and body send.

Notice places in your body where you hold tension, and on a deep breath's exhale, release that tension.

Notice any feelings, positive or negative, that rise to the surface. Take note of them, then let them float away into the darkness.

Notice any messages your body is sending: are you craving something? Coffee or chocolate? Maybe you need a boost of energy. Spinach? Maybe you're a little low on iron or just need some healthy greens. Sunshine and wind? Maybe you've been inside on the couch for a little too long and you need to blow off the stagnation. Take note of those cravings.

When you're ready, take three deep breaths and bring your mind back to the darkness just behind your eyes. Feel your body touching the floor or chair, whether you are cool or warm, and whether there is any remaining tension. Wiggle your toes and fingers and settle back into your physical form.

Open your eyes and start writing down what you made mental notes to remember during your meditation. Don't analyze yet, just write down everything you can think of or remember. Then review the list.

Is your body craving unhealthy food, and is that a craving you want to indulge or curb?

Are you focused on a negative emotion or emotional reaction? What about positive emotions?

Are you ready to let go of some relationship, or job, or lifestyle habit that would bring more balance and peace into your life?

Are you feeling stagnant and ready to find something new to learn or share?

Take some time to think about what you've written down and see which items jump out as most important to you. These are the things that are most unbalanced and may be good to change.

Remember to close your circle, release any guardians or deities you may have called with gratitude, and reground yourself with a snack and some water.

Bibliography and Resources

Campbell, Joseph. *Goddesses, Mysteries of the Feminine Divine*. New World Library, 2013.

—. "Joseph Campbell Quotes." *Goodreads,* www.goodreads.com/author/quotes/20105.Joseph_Campbell

Daimler, Morgan. *The Morrigan: Meeting the Great Queen*. Moon Books, 2012.

—. *Raven Goddess: Going Deeper with The Morrigan*. Moon Books, 2020.

Frankl, Victor. *Man's Search for Meaning*. Beacon Press, 2006.

"Gemstone Meanings & Crystal Properties." *Beadage Healing Jewelry & Gems,* beadage.net/gemstones/

Harris, Stephen L. and Gloria Platzner. *Classical Mythology Images and Insights*. Mayfield Publishing Company, 1995.

"Herbal Grimoire." *The Wiccan Lady,* www.thewiccanlady.co.uk/herbal-grimoire

The Irish Pagan School, irishpaganschool.com/

Jackson, Peter, director. *The Lord of the Rings: The Two Towers*. New Line Cinema, 2002.

Kane, Aurora. *Herbal Magic: A Handbook of Natural Spells, Charms, and Potions*. Quarto Publishing Group, 2021.

Kinsella, Thomas, translator. *The Tain, From the Irish Epic Tain Bo Cúailnge.* Oxford University Press, 1969.

Low, Li Tong. "How a Green Tea Antioxidant Helps Fight Cancer." *Science Connected Magazine*, magazine. scienceconnected.org/2021/03/how-a-green-tea-antioxidant-helps-fight-cancer/

"Magical Properties of Stones and Crystals." *Wiccan Wicca Witchcraft*, wiccanwicca.com/magical-properties-of-stones-and-crystals/

"Magickal Properties of Stones." *Witches of the Craft*, witchesofthecraft.com/2011/12/19/magickal-properties-of-stones/

"Men Leave: Separation and Divorce Far More Common When The Wife Is The Patient." *Science Daily*, https://www.sciencedaily.com/releases/2009/11/091110105401.html

Murphy-Hiscock, Arin. *The Witch's Book of Self-Care.* Adams Media, 2018.

Naim, Raina: *The Art of Letting Go.* Thought Catalog Books, 2016.

O'Brien, Lora. *A Practical Guide to Pagan Priesthood.* Llewellyn Publications, 2019.

Ovid. *Metamorphoses.* Indiana University Press, 1955. Translation by Rolfe Humphries.

Pigliucci, Massimo. *A Field Guide to a Happy Life: 53 Brief Lessons for Living.* Basic Books, 2020.

Skye, Michelle. *Goddess Alive!: Inviting Celtic & Norse Goddesses Into Your Life.* Llewellyn Publications, 2007.

—. *Goddess Afoot!: Practicing Magic with Celtic & Norse Goddesses.* Llewellyn Publications, 2008.

Sobo, Ilana. "Saffron: An Ancient Healing Ally." *The Alchemist's Kitchen*, wisdom.thealchemistskitchen.com/saffron-an-ancient-healing-ally/

Tolkien, J.R.R. *The Fellowship of the Ring.* Houghton Mifflin Company, 1988.

—. Lord of the Rings: *The Two Towers.* Houghton Mifflin, 1956

Toll, Maia. *The Illustrated Herbiary*. Storey Publishing, 2018.
Vaughn, Dan. "Love Lost: The Effects of Cancer on Marriage and Relationships." *Cure*. www.curetoday.com/view/love-lost-the-effects-of-cancer-on-marriage-and-relationships
"Why Does a Breast Cancer Diagnosis Lead to So Many Divorces and Broken Relationships?" *Surviving Breast Cancer*. www.survivingbreastcancer.org/post/why-does-a-breast-cancer-diagnosis-lead-to-so-many-divorces-and-broken-relationships
Wenger, Tibor. "History of Saffron." *Longhua Chinese Medicine*. lcm.amegroups.org/article/view/8189/html#B33
Woodfield, Stephanie. *Priestess of The Morrigan: Prayers, Rituals & Devotional Work to the Great Queen*. Llewellyn Publications, 2021.

CANCER RESOURCES

- American Cancer Society: www.cancer.org
- American Institute for Cancer Research: aicr.org
- Angel Foundation: www.mnangel.org
- Firefly Sisterhood: www.fireflysisterhood.org
- Gilda's Club: www.cancersupportcommunity.org
  - Please note, Gilda's Club is comprised of local chapters, each running their own individual website. All Gilda's Club sites can be found through the Cancer Support Community's website.
- Susan G. Komen Foundation: www.komen.org

Index

A

Abramelin, 25–26
Abundance, 44, 47–49, 94, 123, 181–182, 219, 222, 227, 229, 231–232
Agate, 134, 141
Agency, 27, 38, 160, 168, 172
Allspice, 91, 101
Almond Oil, 77, 92
Aloe Vera, 77, 228
Amber, 142
American Cancer Society, 12, 43
Amethyst, 142
Anger, 38–39, 85, 165, 185
Anise, 101, 108
Aphrodite, 4, 23–24, 38–41
Apollo, 22, 78
Apple, 102, 120
Appropriation, 23–24, 117
Aquamarine, 142
Arnica, 71, 73
Artemis, 83
Asparagus, 120
Avocado, 77, 106, 133

B

Badb, 4, 23, 55, 59–60
Banana, 102, 133
Barley, 102–103
Basil, 47–48, 98, 103, 107, 118, 126, 216, 227
Bay Leaves, 31–32, 103, 124–125, 127, 133, 139, 159–160, 225–226, 233
Beans, 107, 111, 116, 120, 130. See also Legumes
Beltane, 222–224, 226
Bergamot, 130
Bible, 3

Biopsy, 1, 5, 9, 11, 35, 37, 66–67, 147, 167, 182, 201
Black Tourmaline, 134
Blackberry, 103–104, 122–123
Bloodstone, 134, 142–143, 145
Blueberry, 104, 119–120, 122–123, 230–231
Boline, 56, 61
Brigid, 4, 22
Broccoli, 120
Brussels Sprout, 120
Buddhist, 2

C

Calendula, 78
Candle, 4, 18, 25–27, 47–48, 55, 59, 61, 63–65, 72, 84, 89, 92, 133, 135–136, 139, 143–145, 152–154, 159–160, 165, 173–174, 180–182, 184, 192–193, 204–206, 210, 213–214, 219, 224–225, 234
Candle Magic, 139, 173
Caraway, 104
Cardamom, Cardamon, 101, 104
Carrot, 120, 124
Cauliflower, 120
Cedar, 55, 59–60, 89, 91, 95, 97, 213
Celtic, 3, 222
Chakra, 138
Chamomile, 78, 105

Chant, 44, 48, 72, 85, 138, 145, 165–166, 188, 230
Chemo Brain, 104, 119, 163, 191
Chemotherapy, Chemo, 2, 4–6, 20–23, 29–30, 32, 40–42, 46, 53–54, 58, 62, 66, 68–75, 79–81, 85–92, 94, 96, 98, 100–101, 103–107, 109–121, 125, 127–128, 130, 132, 134, 138, 142, 145–146, 148–150, 156, 160–163, 169–172, 179–180, 182, 190–192, 195–196, 205–207, 212, 217–218, 221–222, 225, 227–228, 230, 232–233. See also Radiation
Cherry, 105, 116, 120
Chili, 105–106, 116, 119, 130
Christianity, 2, 21, 57, 155–156
Cinnamon, 48, 91, 93, 101–102, 106, 113, 121–122, 131, 225, 231
Citrine, 44, 94
Cloves, 48–49, 91, 93, 101, 106, 113, 121–122, 126, 131, 225, 231
Coffee, 84, 91, 120, 179, 189, 234
Comfrey, 78
Coriander, 106
Courage, 56, 59, 61–65, 93, 118, 141–143, 145, 203
Cranberry, 107, 120

Cucumber, 107
Cumin, 107, 116

D

Death, 4, 26, 32, 60, 82, 154–155, 167–168, 170–174, 206, 229
Dill, 107, 128
Doxorubicin, 54, 68–69
Dragon's blood, 44–45, 55, 59–60, 90, 93, 181, 213

E

Egyptian, 22
Elderberry, 108
Equinox, 217–218, 221, 232
Eucalyptus, 71–73, 90, 96–97, 108, 112

F

Fennel, 95, 108
Fertility, 102, 107, 168, 219, 222, 227
Firefly Sisterhood, 83
Flax, 95, 108–109
Fluorite, 142
Frankincense, 44–45, 55, 57, 90, 95, 98, 139, 144, 153, 173, 181, 213
Freya, 26
Frigga, 4

G

Gardenia, 98
Garlic, 109, 118, 120, 126–127

Garnet, 142, 207
Gilda's Club, 43, 83, 152
Ginger, 91, 94–95, 101, 106, 109–111, 121–122, 225
Grace, 9, 30, 164–166, 203, 223, 233
Grapefruit, 97–98, 120, 133
Grapes, 120
Grapeseed Oil, 77, 92, 109
Greek, 3, 22, 83, 117
Green Tourmaline, 142
Grief, 168–169, 229, 231–232
Grounding and Centering, 15, 45, 47, 56–58, 62–64, 122, 132, 134–135, 138, 142, 144, 152, 159, 173–174, 181–182, 188, 192–193, 208, 213, 216, 229, 234

H

Hekate, 22
Hematite, 142–144, 192
Hermes, 22
Honey, 84–85, 110–111, 130–131, 181–182
Honeysuckle, 98
Hops, 110

I

Imbolc, 212–213, 215–217
Isis, 22

J

Jade, 44

Jasper, 142–144
Jet, 142, 192
Jewish, 2
Jojoba Oil, 77, 92–93
Juniper, 55, 59–60, 89, 91, 95, 181
Juniper Berry, 55

K
Kale, 120, 124–125, 130

L
Lammas, 229
Lavender, 71–72, 79, 96–97, 231
Legumes, 111, 121. See also Beans; Lentils; Peas
Lemon, 84, 91, 94–95, 97–98, 110–112, 131, 231
Lentils, 111, 120, 123–125. See also Legumes
Lime, 112
Litha, 227
Lughnasadh, 229–232
Lumpectomy, 1, 5, 37, 53, 66, 77, 80, 170
Lymph Node, 37, 53, 66, 162

M
Mabon, 232–234
Macha, 23, 55, 59–60
Magnetic Resonance Imaging (MRI), 5, 35–37, 67, 167, 191, 201

Malachite, 44, 142–143, 145
Marigold, 78
Marinara, 126–127
Marjoram, 127–128
Mastectomy, 1, 37, 53, 66
Meditation, 4–5, 15–18, 25, 27, 84, 87–88, 138, 140, 142, 154, 184, 192, 202, 208, 234–235
Mental Illness, 82
Mesquite, 112
Midsummer, 227–229
Mint, 112, 119. See also Spearmint; Peppermint
Moonstone, 142–143
Morrigan, 4, 23–24, 26, 54–55, 59–60, 83, 92–93, 140, 145, 182, 201–203, 206–207
Moss Agate, 134
Mugwort, 25–26, 55, 60
Muslim, 2
Myrrh, 95
Mythology, 3, 20, 22

N
Nausea, 62, 69, 73–74, 89, 91, 94–95, 100, 109, 112, 114, 118, 171, 185, 206
Neroli, 94, 96
Nettle, 113, 131
Neulasta, 68, 70–71
Neuropathy, 1, 74, 191
Nutmeg, 45–46, 101–102, 106, 113, 131, 225, 231

O

Oatmeal, 104, 106, 109, 113, 119
Oats, 113
Obsidian, 134–135, 143
Offerings, 15, 23, 27, 39, 49, 54–55, 60, 62, 115, 117, 181–182, 207, 217, 220, 231–232
Olive, 95, 109, 113–114, 124, 126–128
Onion, 114, 124, 126–127
Onyx, 142
Orange, 48, 71, 73, 91, 93, 95, 97–98, 106, 114, 120, 133, 231
Oregano, 124–126, 128
Ostara, 217–221, 232–233

P

Panacea, 22
Papaya, 114
Parsley, 96, 115
Patchouli, 45–46
Peach, 122–123
Pea, 111, 120. See also Legumes
Pecan, 122–123
Pepper, 105, 114–115, 124–125, 127–130
Peppermint, 94–95, 98, 112. See also Mint; Spearmint
Persephone, 4, 23–24, 26, 115, 207–208, 210, 221
Plantain, 115
Pomegranate, 115, 130, 207, 209–210
Potato, 100, 115–116, 129–131, 133
Prosperity, 43, 46–47, 102, 106, 113, 118, 121–123
PTSD, 14, 185

Q

Quartz, 134, 143, 145

R

Radiation, 1, 5, 20–21, 30, 32, 42, 53, 62, 75–81, 88, 92, 98, 100, 132, 142, 145–146, 163, 169, 179–180, 184, 190–191, 196, 207, 222, 227–228. See also Chemotherapy, Chemo
Rainbow Moonstone, 142–143
Raspberry, 120
Recurrence, 70, 81, 169, 184, 190, 196, 198–199, 232
Red Devil, The, 54, 69–70, 73–74, 89–90, 105, 138, 161, 163, 218
Ritual, 3–5, 14–15, 19, 23–24, 27, 31–33, 39, 41, 44–45, 47–48, 55–58, 61–65, 68, 71–73, 75, 91–93, 101–102, 109, 113, 116–117, 134, 136, 138–139, 142, 144, 154, 158–160, 165, 181–182, 184, 192–193, 202, 204, 206–207, 213–216, 220, 223–226, 228–231, 233

Rose, 36, 39–41, 98, 143, 145
Rose quartz, 143, 145
Rosemary, 89, 98, 116, 118, 124–125, 127–128, 216, 227, 230

S

Saffron, 117
Sage, 117, 144
Samhain, 201–205, 212
Sandalwood, 98
Sapphire, 143
Sauce, 118, 126–127
Simmer Pot, 48–49
Smoky Quartz, 134
Snowflake Obsidian, 143
Soup, 101–103, 111, 123, 125, 170, 219
Soy, 120, 129
Spearmint, 31–32, 112. See also Mint; Peppermint
Spinach, 120, 130, 234
Squash, 120
Strawberry, 120, 228, 231
Surgery, 1, 5, 20–21, 28–30, 32, 37–38, 40–42, 53, 66, 68, 80–81, 93, 145, 156, 179–180, 182, 190
Susan G. Komen Foundation, 2, 12, 43

T

Talisman, 118, 141, 146, 152–153, 180
Tarragon, 128

Taxol, 73–75, 92, 105, 119–120, 163, 170–171, 218
Tea, 63, 71, 78, 84–85, 94, 97, 101, 104–106, 108–113, 118–120, 130–131, 226
Tea Tree, 97
Tea, Black, 84, 106, 118, 131
Tea, Green, 71, 84, 110, 130–131
Therapist, 83, 147, 164, 184, 186, 189, 195, 198, 232
Therapy, 82–84, 152, 185–186, 199, 227
Thor, 26
Thyme, 93–95, 98, 116, 118, 124–125, 128, 216, 230
Tiger's Eye, 44, 63–64, 94, 134, 143
Tomato, 107, 118, 120, 126–127
Tumor, 11, 21, 28, 37, 53, 66–67, 81, 145, 162, 169
Turmeric, 115, 119, 130–131

U

Ultrasound, 5, 10–11, 35, 67, 201
Unverified Personal Gnosis (UPG), 23–24

V

Vanilla, 98, 129

W

Walnut, 119–120
Whole Grain, 113, 120

Wicca, Wiccan, 3–4, 136, 201, 229
Wintergreen, 119
Witch Hazel, 79, 97

Y

Yarrow, 94
Yew, 74, 119–120
Ylang-Ylang, 98
Yule, 80, 115, 149, 156, 205–207, 212